Cancer and the Philosophy of the Far East

George Ohsawa

George Ohsawa Macrobiotic Foundation
Chico, California

Other books by George Ohsawa in English include: *The Art of Peace; Essential Ohsawa; Gandhi, the Eternal Youth; Jack and Mitie; Macrobiotic Guidebook for Living; Macrobiotics: An Invitation to Health and Happiness; Order of the Universe; Philosophy of Oriental Medicine; The Unique Principle; You Are All Sanpaku;* and *Zen Macrobiotics.* Contact the publisher at the address below for a complete list of available titles.

In memory of Al Brand

Keyboarding by Alice Salinero
Proofreading/editing by Kathy Keller
Text layout and design by Carl Ferré
Cover design by Carl Campbell

First English Edition	1971
First G.O.M.F. Edition	1981, 1984
Current Printing: edited and reformatted	2012 Sep 1

Published with the help of East West Center for Macrobiotics
   www.eastwestmacrobiotics.com

Library of Congress Catalog Card Number: 78-159569
ISBN 978-0-918860-69-9

Publisher's Preface

I am taking the opportunity to publish this preface because of misunderstandings that have arisen about George Ohsawa's writings.

In his lifetime, George Ohsawa tried to unite religious and cultural organizations (such as "Ito-En," "Chushin-Kai," "Japanese Women's Federation," "Japanese Yoga Association," "Seicho-No-Ie," etc.) that were interested in macrobiotic philosophy.

In December 1963, he gathered these foremost Japanese spiritual, cultural, and medical leaders together for a meeting in Tokyo. At this meeting, he asked them to compile advice on healing for the Western World. The result of that idea materialized into this book, but it ended up as solely George Ohsawa's writing instead of the compilation of many writings that he had hoped for.

Ohsawa learned both Oriental and Western approaches to health; he is one of the few who knew both the shortcomings of Western medicine and the advantages of Oriental medicine. Therefore, in this book, he is offering advice on the cure of cancer from the Oriental medical point of view. However, this is not the cancer cure book that most people would imagine, but rather it is a spiritual book on how to overcome the fear of incurable diseases, of which cancer is one.

On June 30, 1982, the Los Angeles Times published an article called "Perhaps Cancer Can Be a State of Mind," written by Colman McCarthy. In this article he writes: "At a recent New York Academy of Medicine Conference, Dr. Joan Borysenko, speaking on 'fear, hope, and cancer,' said that there is considerable data that points to an influence of behavioral factors on the course of a disease. Hopelessness, helplessness, and fear correlate with decreased survival. These emotions are associated with hormonal changes that depress the activity of the immune system. The preservation of hope, the determination to fight the disease, and the will to live are correlated with enhanced survival and improved quality of life."

Recently, the medical healing establishment has begun taking into account the patient's mind and behavior, as well as diet, along with conventional treatment. However, in the medical field today very few know how to preserve a patient's hope, faith in a cure, or will to live. Contrary to Western medicine, Oriental medicine developed ways of improving the mentality and behavior of patients.

Eastern culture developed spiritually, while Western culture developed somewhat materialistically. The former developed understanding of mind and spirit. The latter developed wealth, technology, and science. Western medicine, therefore, generally takes the materialistic approach to the curing of sickness. Western medicine's methods of cancer cure are cutting, burning, and poisoning. Those methods do not show much success. One of the reasons Western medicine cannot succeed at curing cancer lies in the fact that cancer creates fear, mental instability, and psychological problems. To these situations, Eastern medicine can make a contribution, because Eastern religion (such as Buddhism) established a psychological approach to illness.

George Ohsawa is presenting in this book the spiritual cure for sickness, and especially cancer. I believe that someone who is suffering from fear, as well as uncertainty, will be able to benefit by reading this book repeatedly. George Ohsawa said in this book, "In order to cure a cancer patient who has already surrendered, it is first necessary to change his attitude. This must be accomplished at any cost." That attitude that must change is revealed in this book. This is a book of spiritual healing.

Herman Aihara
July 1984

Contents

I am very happy that this materialization of Mr. Ohsawa's wonderful book has at last become a reality, and I want to express my heartfelt thanks to the many people who have contributed their knowledge, time, and energy to its completion. I am particularly indebted to Armand la Belle and Ralph Baccash, who translated it from the French, and to Lou Oles, Lennie Richards, and Bill French, who devoted many long and painstaking hours to revising and re-revising the contents.

I sincerely hope that this book will help us all to understand and practice the order of man.

Herman Aihara, President
George Ohsawa Macrobiotic Foundation

Author's Letter of Introduction
Paris, 1963

Dear Friends of all Countries,

I have written this book at the beginning of my seventy-second year, still following the same path I have walked alone for fifty years. My aim in this, my seventh work in French, is as always to produce mutual understanding between East and West. I want to help you understand the mentality of the Orientals and other colonized peoples whom Lèvy-Bruhl has called "primitive." The way things are going today, this mentality should soon disappear. Primitive people everywhere are nearing extinction or assimilation by the "civilized," after the manner of the American Indian.

The primitive mentality is without doubt simple, childlike, and, sometimes, even ridiculous. But it possesses something that is very beautiful, very practical, and very profound. Unknown among civilized people, this precious jewel is an extremely simple dialectical philosophy condensed into two antagonistic words: Yin and Yang, Tamas and Rajas, etc. This philosophy, a synthetical [Ed. note: based on synthesis or unification; opposed to "analytical" or differentiated.] understanding of the world, is the wellspring and unifying force of all sciences and techniques of the Far East. Oriental medicine, for example, is only one application of this Unifying Principle according to which all phenomena appear to us as opposites.

Dialectical monism was also well known in Europe, even two thousand years before Christ, among the Druids and the Celts. In fact, it has never been totally destroyed even in modern times. The principal agent of its decline has been the manner in which the religion of Jesus, Christianity, has been interpreted. That is to say, it has been rendered absolutely dualistic (meaning two natures: Good

and Evil, God and the Devil, Material and Spiritual, Soul and Body).
St. Thomas Aquinas, for example, was a fanatical dualist: "In this
world," he claimed, "there can never be too much good." This is a
wholly artificial view.

Hegel, however, studied and taught this paradoxical monistic
dialectic. Then Karl Marx, a student of Hegel, made use of the principle to strengthen his own sociological theory. His followers, in
turn, have succeeded in establishing a powerful society based on
dialectical logic. The modern-day result has been the development
of the world's first Sputniks.

But no one has yet discovered the way to apply this dialectic to
the science of life. In the West, biology, biochemistry, physiology,
and medicine have failed to penetrate to the essence of life. They
study only the structure of the living, utilizing physical and chemical observations, which stop at the level of the electron. Yet Life
(Oneness) is far more profound than this. It creates the nuclei of all
atoms as well as all organisms capable of transmuting these atoms.
Life transmutes atoms without requiring either great heat or pres-
sure. Is this not miraculous? And it creates, above all, the mental and
spiritual activities such as imagination, comprehension, judgment,
will, and thought.

The philosophy of the Far East, unifier of biology, biochemistry,
physiology, agriculture, botany, zoology, and medicine, teaches us
how to cure all illnesses declared "incurable" by Western medicine;
and this by a method sometimes called "paradoxical"—that is, without bloody operations, using no chemical products, and functioning solely through the simple choice of daily foods. This method is
known as macrobiotics.

Many of you have seen it work. Its practice has cured great numbers who had been declared "incurable" by official medicine. Some
of you have taught it and have saved many others so that today most
health-food and large department stores in France, Belgium, and the
United States carry macrobiotic (locally grown, whole) foods. Yet,
official medicine continues to ignore the appearance of macrobiotics,
even though it *has* recognized the utility and effectiveness of acu-

puncture, which I introduced to the West more than thirty-five years ago. Undoubtedly, this is due to the fact that acupuncture is a symptomatic treatment, so simple to learn that one can apply it without having to study the Unifying Principle in depth. (Massage and moxa are equally symptomatic, easy to learn, and practical.) There are tens of thousands of practicing acupuncturists in Japan, hundreds of thousands in China, and at least five thousand in Europe (mainly in France and Germany). In 1956, it was widely discussed in all the Parisian newspapers. And, recently, an extensive article called "A Different Medicine: Acupuncture" appeared in the magazine *Planète* (Number 13).

Flower arrangement, Judo, and Bonsai (natural miniature landscaping)—applications of the Unifying Principle of Yin and Yang that I began demonstrating in Paris forty years ago—are widespread today. Above all, rice cultivation, which was completely absent from France forty years ago, is now a major agricultural enterprise. Today, France is one of the largest producers of rice in Europe—100,000,000 kilos per year. [Ed. note: one kilo equals about two pounds.] One can buy it everywhere, even in 50-kilo sacks. Forty years ago, however, rice was sold only in two-ounce boxes! I was forced to buy about a hundred boxes a month! How difficult it was to find a grocer able to satisfy me...

But everything changes. Time marches on. There are now five macrobiotic restaurants in Paris where one can eat whole ("brown") rice, as well as others in New York, Los Angeles, and even Stockholm: Viking country!

Why then doesn't official Western medicine recognize and recommend macrobiotics? Could it be that it is avoiding loss of face?

At any rate, because official medicine is helpless before cancer, it is now considered by Western man as his greatest enemy. Yet, according to the dialectical philosophy of Eternal Happiness and Absolute Freedom, cancer is in reality a profound benefactor of mankind. It is cancer that slows down the catastrophic speed of our civilization—which is hurrying pell-mell toward the very extremities of dualism!

While hydrogen bombs restrain us from totally annihilating one another, cancer saves us from the dead end of scientific and technical materialism—a stranger to life, to spirituality, to the world itself, and to the Absolute Justice that creates and governs everything, everywhere.

You have already seen sick people who have cured themselves by studying and practicing this dialectical philosophy, in Europe as well as in the United States. Often, they had been officially declared "incurable," not only of cancer but of all sorts of physical and mental diseases as well. And what is more, they have attained what men have sought for thousands of years: Eternal Happiness (awareness of the Absolute Justice of all that ever happens, any time, anywhere).

The aim of all the great religions of man has been, it seems to me, to teach the individual how to overcome his physical and mental sufferings; that is to say, how to attain health, longevity, and emotional control, which are the fundamental bases of human happiness and freedom.

But through the centuries, religions have fallen into the hands of professionals who are nothing but phonographs reciting sacred words. Some scholars, it is true, possess conceptual knowledge of the aims of religion but, unfortunately, they remain impractical.

Having spent more than fifty years studying and teaching the Unifying Principle, I believe that the time has come to address myself to Occidental thinkers, asking them to study this paradoxical logic, childlike and apparently "too simple," yet in reality very practical and effective when applied to daily life. Such is my purpose in writing this little book.

It is now generally recognized that our scientific and technological civilization, if not all of humanity, is on the brink of catastrophe! Modern civilized man is engulfed in dark clouds of uncertainty; of political, sociological, and physiological fear; of fear of crime and "incurable" disease, the most deadly of which is cancer.

Civilized people have, without doubt, succeeded in revolutionizing this world of slavery and misery and in establishing a brilliant scientific and technical base without equal or precedent in the entire history of mankind. We all admire and cherish it.

But "the bigger the front, the bigger the back." This brilliant civilization, and with it all of humanity, are threatened from moment to moment with extinction. We can reduce ourselves to dust!

What a pity!

But what is the cause of this potential self-annihilation?

Scientific, technological civilization, gigantic and extremely powerful in its apparent scope, plunges onward with ever-increasing speed, constantly accelerating through the darkness of an unknown sea. The crew of this huge ocean liner mobilizes all its precision instruments in an effort to chart a safe course. But alas, the instruments do not provide the hoped-for results. The entire crew is exhausted and desperate...

Among the millions of passengers on this liner is an old Oriental who knows how to point a safe passage, according to a constellation of far-distant stars. He willingly offers his knowledge of an ancient astronomy that, according to Bios the Elder and Bios the Younger, could predict solar eclipses four thousand years ago! However, his astronomy is not all that this old passenger has to offer; he would also like to show you a way of life that is capable of changing all unhappiness into happiness. In fact, this old traveler can affirm that the greater the unhappiness, the greater the happiness that is reached in overcoming it!

In conclusion, let me say that all your criticisms, no matter how informal, will be received with great joy. I am entirely at your disposal and will gladly furnish you with any information you wish concerning this philosophy-physiology of the Far-East.

Does Dr. Schweitzer Represent the Western Mentality?

Leave immediately, immediately!

This dictatorial, maddening command still resounds in my ears, even though many years have passed since I heard it. At that time, I was in Lambaréné, South Africa, having arrived there with my wife by plane via Brazzaville in October, 1955. I had been given a brotherly welcome by Miss Emma, a collaborator of Dr. Schweitzer's. Although industrious and courageous, she was in poor physiological condition, having gained much weight.

Lambaréné is a small hospital village with a population of approximately seven hundred, of whom about forty are white. These comprise the staff of the hospital, all others being patients. My wife, Jotsuna (Ed. note: name given to Mr. Ohsawa's wife, Lima, in India; meaning "moon") worked every day in the kitchen with black cooks and a white girl, all of whom perspired enormously and drank copiously. In spite of the intense African heat, my wife remained cool and calm. I leave it to your imagination how hot it was. The moist air steamed under a torrid sun. Everyone retired early and required an afternoon nap. One avoided going out—even in the evening. Yet I was able to work an average of twenty hours a day, starting at 2 a.m. by the light of a kerosene lamp.

Lambaréné is a true paradise. The natives have no agriculture. They fish in the great river or hunt in the jungle for monkeys, boa, wild boar, and elephant. After a wild manioc dinner (manioc is a kind of sweet potato), they go to bed immediately because they possess neither electricity nor gas. For them, life is a continual round of hunting or fishing. They do not know the meaning of work—they only know how to have fun. Poor but indifferent to their poverty, they live in a real paradise.

But I have seen the other side of this paradise. "Bigger the front, bigger the back." The greater the ease, the greater the hardship. *Any paradise in this relative world has a reverse aspect.* And I have lived through both paradise and hell in Lambaréné: the most terrible hell in this world.

Flaming green and great, the river flows on night and day, noiselessly, so broad that half an hour is required to cross it by canoe, so rapid that it cannot be traversed perpendicularly.

At the hospital we eat with the forty white staff members. The food that they (and I, but not Jotsuna) eat is terrible, consisting mainly of honey, black molasses, jam, coffee or tea with powdered milk, sugar, and large amounts of fruit. Everything except the fruit is imported from Europe. Little by little one consumes two to four pounds of sugar per month. At lunch and dinner, the food is "à l'Alsacienne", accompanied by mangoes, papayas, bananas, and coconuts, all of which were introduced about thirty years ago and, therefore, cannot be considered staples in this area. Also, the occasional use of pastries further increases the destructive imbalance.

I accept everything that is given to me except sugar, honey, jam and the most yin condiments. After a few weeks I begin to experience pain: toothache, stiff neck, eye fatigue, diarrhea, urethritis, discomfort in the kidneys; it becomes worse and worse every day.

My wife maintains a simple macrobiotic eating pattern, avoiding sugar and animal products completely and limiting her intake of fruits to a very small amount.

She eats five to six ounces of white rice and approximately one ounce of salad or two ounces of vegetables cooked with salt as daily food. Her liquid intake is limited to about one glass of water a day.

Except for sugar, I eat like the whites. But, I walk bareheaded and barefoot like the blacks.

The whites are protected by tropical helmets, shoes, and stockings (some double-layered) filled with iodoform (an antiseptic-disinfectant iodine compound). Moreover, they take pills. Everyone reprimands me because I walk barefooted, shun a helmet, and refuse pills. But, I cannot be shielded like the whites while millions of Africans go barefoot or remain half-naked. They are poor; their food costs one-tenth of that of whites. So, if they cannot be provided with a tropical helmet, shoes, and several pairs of stockings, then I too must walk barefoot and bareheaded. I must show the whites that one can retain good health and cure any disease without artificial instruments in this tropical African climate.

I want to eat as the natives do, but this is impossible. They have an extremely strict tabu, never sharing food or eating what has been prepared by others. This way of living is ideal, physically and morally. All year long their staple is manioc. Only in January do they eat green bananas, which are bitter and astringent and completely unlike the sweet bananas reserved "for the whites." The remainder of their diet consists of 5% to 10% wild herbs and 2% to 3% meat (monkey, boa, elephant, antelope, and dried or smoked fish). They eat little fruit because plantations are non-existent, and fruit in its wild state is scarce in the jungle. (Being relatively low in calories, fruit cannot serve as a source of staple nourishment anyway.) Eating large amounts of fruit is beyond reach of the poor natives, who simply gather what falls in the jungle.

Because there are no wells or springs and the river is contaminated with hospital refuse of pus and blood, they drink rain water. Their diet stands in direct opposition to that of the colonizers, whose menu contains more than two hundred items, while the natives restrict themselves to only five or six of which 80% to 90% is manioc. Thus, the blacks are very macrobiotic! For although manioc is very yin, *it can be considered a balanced food in such a yang climate*. The natives should be in brilliant health and, indeed, they are. The Bantus, for example, whose diet is extremely limited compared to the Europeans' and Americans', are incomparably more healthy than both. (From Dr. A.R.P. Walker's report to the "Nutrition Conference" organized by the New York Academy of Sciences in Johannesburg, March, 1957.)

Most Gabonese also were, and still are, as healthy and strong as the Bantus. Some, however, who have been "civilized" by Westerners and take wine, sugar, and sweetened condensed milk from France, are degenerating. Before Western explorer-colonizers penetrated the interior of Africa, all natives were healthy, much more than the colonizers themselves in their own country. They enjoyed living in the vast jungle, free of laws imposed by the strongest. They were peaceful, honest, courageous, and amiable; they accepted everything that was given, and gave everything that was asked. If you wish to verify this, read Stanley's *Black Africa* or the works of Dr. Livingstone.

Like Asians, Africans give everything and accept everything—their resources, land, products, labor, even their country. They are prepared to abandon their own traditions, so it is not only their fault but also that of the West if they have lost their original characteristics. (Please read Lèvy-Bruhl's *Primitive Mentality*.)

The Gabonese, as well as all Africans, have been and would still be happy, healthy, and amiable if the whites had not imported alcohol and capitalistic, industrialized sugar. They knew nothing of diseases such as leprosy. Incredible as it may seem, I have cured a great number of Africans suffering from so-called "incurable" diseases simply by suppressing alcohol, sugar, and sweets from their diet. This appeared "miraculous" to them, and the number of patients visiting me increased steadily. When I left the hospital, several blacks bid me good-bye with tears in their eyes. And while I lived at the Protestant Mission, a little more than a mile from the hospital, the number of patients who came to consult me increased even more. There were many who traveled several hundred miles by canoe each day. I felt obliged to say that I could no longer receive them, for I was afraid that all the patients would come to me instead of going to Dr. Schweitzer's hospital. (Ed. note: This is a good example of a fundamental difference between the Eastern and Western mentalities. Had Schweitzer asked him, Ohsawa would have been glad to help as many patients as possible. But because they were already going to

Schweitzer, Ohsawa would not want to intrude by soliciting them to come to him—even though he was quite sure that his advice would be more helpful than Schweitzer's.)

Those of you who know the Unifying Principle can imagine how dangerous it is for a foreigner to eat like the "civilized," shun protection for his head, and prefer walking barefoot in the African jungle. In this extremely hot and humid country of luxuriant vegetation, molds, bacteria, viruses, and all sorts of small yin insects such as flies, mosquitoes, lice, and ants multiply abundantly. Walking barefoot in the jungle is like navigating on torpedoes: filaria, chiggers, spirochetes... This is a real hellhole of disease where one is "attacked" by microscopic beings.

During the second month, my general condition worsened, especially the urethritis. Of course, the cause was European food accompanied by so much extremely yin tropical fruit. Europeans are incapable of remaining in Africa for several years—in spite of their precautions and medications. Even Dr. Schweitzer does not remain there constantly. The courageous staff members of the hospital, most of whom are women (only four or five men), with a few exceptions do not remain longer than two years at a time. Nearly all are more or less ailing, the two physicians being most seriously afflicted.

Finally, I am assaulted simultaneously by filaria, chiggers, and the spirochetes of tropical ulcers, which are a thousand times more terrible than leprosy. The filaria parasite attacks my head, causing my face to grow swollen and deformed. Strangely enough, no pain results. But chiggers settle under my nails and lay hundreds of eggs, which cause very painful wounds.

The spirochetes penetrate the skin everywhere and produce several one-inch tumors that eventually grow to over a foot in length and nearly an inch in depth. They are filled with a violet-black liquid. When these tumors are lanced, very deep cavities are seen, sometimes baring white bone. Blood, pus, and liquid discharged from the cavities are insulting, repulsive. A nauseating smell fills the room. The pain is unbearable. In four or five weeks, death comes, the body a mass of sores. With leprosy, one can sometimes survive for twenty or even thirty years, and there is no pain. But with tropical ulcers, the reality of the disease is beyond description. (If you wish to learn more, read pages 209 to 211 of *Tropical Medicine* by Dr. Clement Chesterman, ex-manager of the Baptist Hospital, Republic of the Congo.)

I had fasted during the months of August and September, 1955, while traveling from Dar–es–Sa-laam—via Mombassa, Nairobi, Kampala, and Stanleyville—to Leopoldville, a distance of approximately 3,000 miles. Continually caring for patients en route, I was quite weak upon arrival at Lambaréné in October. The very highly yin hospital food weakened me, because I had not yet fully recovered from the sixty days of fasting, but I never ceased working.

January 4, 1955: I am attacked by chiggers in my small right toe. Very painful. I continue working day and night.

January 11: The pain increases and becomes unbearable. I cannot go on typing the manuscript of *The Philosophy of Far Eastern Medicine*.

I abandon my work and lie down as Jotsuna asks me to. It is 8 p.m. and I must finish my work, at the latest, before the evening of the 13th.

In bed, the pain increases. Cramps grip my neck, hands, and legs. Could it be tetanus? Three afternoons ago, while everybody was napping, I cleaned the mud behind the kitchen. It was very dirty. Then, still working barefooted, I cleaned the garden. Can this be tetanus?

My little finger has swollen to twice its normal size and is violet-colored. The pain grows more and more intense. I must lance the toe, but with what? Must I ask Dr. P. to operate? But the hospital is far away. Jotsuna cannot go there all by herself. It is past midnight. Nobody can ferry her upstream by canoe against the fast river. Must I wait until morning? Too long! And then what can I do in the morning?

Oh, how painful! For more than four hours I toss and turn. I cannot remain motionless for even an instant. I am going insane!

Jotsuna prepares a black poultice of "dentie" (burnt eggplant and unrefined salt) and covers my toe. I submit helplessly, having no idea what to do.

Strangely enough, I fall asleep. Is it out of fatigue or because the pain is disappearing?

Whenever I am suffering, I go to bed. Such is my habit. I lose consciousness immediately because I sleep only four hours a day. I can always fall asleep anywhere, in two or three minutes. And, when I sleep my pain disappears immediately. Sleeping is my catch-all remedy. I think that sleeping more than six hours a day is laziness. God works night and day. If the Son of God allowed himself to sleep at all, it was only for one-sixth or one-seventh of his working time— no more. Once, eight years ago, I tried to do completely without sleep and managed to work thus for fifty-seven days, translating an extremely difficult English book, *The Meeting of East and West*, by Professor F.C.S. Northrup. The original text contained 500 pages; my manuscript 2,000. Of course, I maintained a very special diet (a very yang one) during that period. When I was twenty, I slept from 9 p.m. to 3 a.m.; at fifty, from 10 p.m. to 2 a.m. as a rule; after the age of seventy, I hope to sleep even less.)

January 12: I awaken at 2 a.m. I feel no pain. Has the tetanus disappeared? I jump out of bed to catch up with my work. But I cannot walk without pain.

At 6 a.m., Jotsuna awakens and is stunned to see me at my writing table. Neither of us has guessed that the pain of the previous day was but the prelude to the dreadful onset of tropical ulcers.

A beautiful day breaks at Lambaréné. In spite of the low roof, light penetrates our shabby room in the old cottage where Dr. Schweitzer began his work more than forty years ago. I examine the toe that so tormented me yesterday. Jotsuna begs me not to touch it. It has tripled in size and is as taut as a balloon. I puncture it with a needle. Dirty liquid spurts out, bringing relief. But I still cannot stand or walk. The weight of my body expands the swollen capillaries of my right leg until they feel as though they might burst.

I cover my swollen, sensitive toe with a large blade of grass, then don a slipper for concealment. Walking on my heel, I painfully cross the garden to breakfast in the big house with the minister and his family. With difficulty, I climb to the second floor. The priest and his wife ask if there is something wrong.

"It's nothing," I reply, "just a little wound."

But I am terribly mistaken.

January 13: A dozen new balloon-like tumors appear. I puncture, salt, and rub them. Very painful. A boil has arisen on the old tumor. I remove it and expose a cavity.

Is this a typical disease of the country? The symptoms are mysterious and unknown to me.

A great deal of work remains to be done. I am in a hurry. I must finish this evening and spend the night reading over the manuscript before presenting it early tomorrow to Dr. Schweitzer as a birthday gift.

From 9 a.m. until noon and from 2 to 5 in the afternoon, I must attend to black patients as usual. I work frantically. Jotsuna is busy washing old napkins and disposing of Japanese newspapers, soaked with pus and blood, which I have employed as dressings.

January 15: I ask a black student from the mission school to take my book, *The Philosophy of Far Eastern Medicine*, to Dr. Schweitzer. I am finished with my 90-day effort.

Time passes. Every day, new tumors. The toes on both feet are bulbous. Feet, legs, arms, and hands are covered with boils and tumors. The room is bilious with a nauseating stench.

During the day, black patients beseech me. Also I must write and read. But my urethritis worsens, and I urinate every two hours. Three times a day, I must go to the big house for my meals.

The weather grows increasingly warmer. It is the dry season. From time to time, the two lady teachers invite us for dinner and the black instructors ask for lectures on philosophy and medicine in the evenings. Jotsuna busies herself revolutionizing the kitchen in the minister's house. His entire family is ill. He himself suffers from heart disease and falling hair; his wife, who is hospitalized from time to time, is very irritable, nervous, and fatigued; his eldest daughter, who is seven, suffers from eye trouble; the second, who is five, has poliomyelitis; and the youngest, only four months old, lacks appetite, spitting up her condensed milk and crying continually.

Stupefaction! Amazement! I discover that I am beset with—*tropical ulcers!* I am to die within a few weeks! One week has already passed... But I must confirm the symptoms and conditions described by Dr. Chesterman in *Tropical Medicine*. I cannot cure a disease without knowing in detail all its aspects. How else could I be qualified to attend to my black friends?

Second week: My condition worsens dismally.

Third week...

Fourth week: My body is devoured by pain. I can no longer sleep, nor can I care for patients. Walking is impossible. I am nothing but a gnawed, half-buried corpse, hollowed and deformed by invisible germs. My body is a mass of rotting flesh, oozing pus and blood, and emitting a noxious, foul smell. All my toe-nails have fallen out.

January 28: Near midnight, a big rat gnaws at my foot, mistaking it for a piece of decaying meat.

It is time to start rescuing myself. Otherwise, rats will devour both my legs while snakes and boas come to swallow the remainder. I can hear them in the night.

But I must not die! I have millions and millions of black brothers and sisters to save!

Tropical ulcers being an extremely yin disease, one has to decrease all that is yin through proper diet. The food at the Protestant Mission is even poorer than the hospital's; although, since January 1, Jotsuna has changed the diet of the minister's household. Unfortunately, whole rice is unavailable. She sends schoolboys through the poor local rice paddies gathering rice, grain by grain. But a whole day is required to collect only a small amount.

We possess no normal foodstuffs. Canoeing up or down the river to the neighboring village would take at least half a day, only to find some sweetened preserves and potatoes imported from France at the other end.

Nothing else.

Fortunately, unexpectedly, a small packet arrives from New York by air. One of my former girl students (Cornellia Aihara) has sent me two pounds of roasted brown rice and a few "umeboshi" (Japanese plums preserved in salt for one year or more). Yang accompanies yin—every cloud has a silver lining. Suffering is nothing but the beginning of joy.

I decide to save myself in ten days. What would you have done in my place? How would you have accomplished it?

Picture yourself in the jungle. No grocery stores, no running water, no electricity. Jot down your answer immediately on a sheet of paper, then read what follows.

January 29: I decide to stop drinking water completely, not even one drop. I shall have one glass of roasted brown rice instead.

At night, Jotsuna pours about three ounces of rice into an ordinary glass and adds a small amount of boiling water. By morning, the liquid has evaporated, and I eat it with an "umeboshi." That is all for the day. Before retiring at night, I take a few ounces of salt. (Salt is a necessary component in the K/Na [Potassium/Sodium] balance of our bodies.) And I do not drink at all. Nothing else.

Jotsuna, too, is ill. Every other day she removes hundreds of chigger eggs from under her nails. She has also contracted tropical ulcers, two or three having appeared on her hands. But Dr. Chesterman's *Tropical Medicine* states that women are immune to this disease. Do you understand why his viewpoint is wrong?

From February 1st through 3rd, I am completely immobilized and think of many things. Oh, how happy I would be if someone would only send me a parcel of *tekka* or *miso*. It is extremely difficult to assimilate salt, which, if introduced in large amounts into the intercellular (between the cells) channels, is insufficient to modify the levels of intracellular (within cells) potassium. Besides, ingesting so much raw salt is very painful.

Oh, tekka! Miso! Kimpira!

So many thoughts cross my mind. I write a hundred pages in Japanese as if composing my last will. A pity I have never had time to translate them.

After all, if you have not suffered the pain and agony of tropical ulcers, if you have not been covered with pus and blood and been gnawed by a rat, if you have not been overwhelmed by the foul smell of your own putrefying flesh, then you are not able to say whether you sympathize with or have any compassion for black Africans. Dr. Schweitzer realizes this.

Avoiding the consequences of the disease through artificial means would be cowardly. This is not the way of a sincere man, especially a "samurai." One must see the disease through and overcome it without killing. The germs, in other words, must be allowed to live peacefully. Killing to defend oneself is not just.

Since January 30, no new tumors have appeared. The ulcers are drying up day by day. The pain is disappearing. The disease is overcome. It has stopped. The germs are leaving my body peacefully. *How wise they are!*

On February 4, at 4 p.m., a loud voice echoes through the jungle: "Great Doctor! Great Doctor!"

I climb out of bed. In the distance, a canoe can be seen on the river. It is Dr. Schweitzer himself. But I cannot even go down to the beach to welcome him, for the slope is too steep and long.

Everyone converges on the beach—schoolboys, schoolgirls, the minister and his wife. African lepers guide the canoe to land, and the great doctor and his wife step ashore.

What a shame! I cannot even leave my cottage!

The great doctor enters and commands:

"Show me your ulcers!"

"It is nothing, Dr. Schweitzer."

"Show me your ulcers!"

I cannot escape. I exhibit my right foot, which is less afflicted—or, rather, more relieved.

The doctor wordlessly scrutinizes my foot. He does not touch it.

"You must leave immediately," he declares.

"Can it not be cured, Dr. Schweitzer?"

"Impossible. Leave immediately."

Stunned, I am speechless. I search for words, but in vain...

"May I not—."

"Impossible!" he interrupts in a louder voice. "Leave immediately!"

"But you could teach me how to cure this disease, couldn't you?"

"No. It is impossible. Besides, you can't stay here any longer. The mission is poor."

"But I came here to teach how to cure this disease through—"

"No. Impossible. You know nothing about this disease. You think you have learned a lot here. But what you have learned is nothing compared to what you still do not know. Africa is vast. You'll have to leave immediately."

Each time I begin to speak, my words, my voice are crushed, overwhelmed. I cannot go on. I do the best I can.

"But I must—recover—"

"Impossible. Leave immediately! LEAVE IMMEDIATELY!"

"Is there no way, Dr. Schweitzer?"

"No! It's impossible!"

"Good! Then I will cure mys—"

"No! IMPOSSIBLE! LEAVE! There is nothing to be done. You have failed to observe my prescriptions from the very beginning. You were supposed to wear double-thick stockings filled with iodoform."

He sermonizes. Being very yin by birth, I remain silent, listening. A long sermon... Each time I try to interject a comment, I am overwhelmed. I wish to tell him that it is our duty to teach millions upon millions of Africans how to maintain the superb health their forefathers enjoyed, without medication, and how to cure themselves, because they are poor, without recourse to expensive drugs. But, this is out of the question. I want to warn the doctor that all or almost all the Africans I have met either at the hospital or outside the compound are more or less against him. They are suspicious and rebellious because the number of patients constantly increases. Once hospitalized, patients are not freed for the rest of their lives. Instead, maimed, mutilated, limbs amputated, they remain prisoners. Several have been hospitalized for more than three, five, or seven years. They can no longer get out.

In vain. There is nothing I can do with my poor knowledge of French.

As he exits, the doctor repeats, "Leave immediately."

But first, I answer silently, I must cure myself. I cannot walk— but do I really have to go? I came to Lambaréné to explain to him the medicine of the Far East, for he is considered "The Man of the Century." He is the supreme pacifist. He insists upon reverence for life. If he can comprehend the Unifying Principle and the Order of the Universe, he can possibly save the world. I must give him everything. Yes, if he wants me and asks me, I will remain here all my life...

In order to fulfill this dream, I had come to Lambaréné after coping with untold hardships, risking my life on many occasions, and spending thousands of dollars.

But now I was depressed and lonely, thoroughly dejected. At that moment, Jotsuna spoke.

"Impossible? Many times he said a cure was impossible. Is he right?"

"You heard him?"

"Yes. So all we have to do is recover completely. He will see. He'll want to know how we cured this 'incurable' disease, and he'll understand. Hasn't he read your book?"

"Yes. He said he had read it all."

"Well then, hasn't he criticized it?"

"He hasn't understood, it seems to me, judging by his attitude and the things he said."

"Then we'll have to show him our complete recovery! These tropical ulcers are nothing. You feel better and so do I. Why can't we cure them? 'All visible and invisible phenomena have a beginning *and* an end,' remember? We just have to cure ourselves and let the evidence convince him. If he doesn't understand your French, at least he'll understand your recovery. You haven't lost your courage, have you?"

"No. And you're right. The evidence will convince him."

"The hospital workers haven't understood, and they aren't even interested in our medicine and philosophy. But surely the Great Doctor will understand. He must understand. And when he understands, we'll work here, all our lives. I'll work in the kitchen with the patients. Already they're wondering about me, beginning to look at me curiously as if asking themselves how I can work so long without perspiring or getting tired."

The minister enters. He has been instructed to get rid of us as quickly as possible. "Leave immediately," he says.

"I beg you, dear Mr. M., wait another week. I'll show you a miracle—then I'll leave forever."

He does not insist, because his entire family has already been saved. His wife no longer shouts—her nervous voice has ceased chattering and echoing through the wide jungle, and the instructors and students are very happy about that. Even Mr. D., the school manager, has mentioned the change. The minister, meanwhile, has stopped losing his hair and his fatigue has disappeared. Most important, his three little girls have improved. Françoise is better behaved; Anne has lost her morose clumsiness and, instead, sings cheerfully; and the youngest, Christine, who continually rejected sweetened milk, has emptied in one sitting her first bottle of milk and brown (whole) rice. She does not cry anymore, has a pleasant disposition, and sleeps well. She smiles whenever my wife nears her and, more than once, has moistened Jotsuna's dress with her urine...

The minister withdraws politely, doubtful that he will witness a "miracle"—but at least he is prepared to wait for a few days.

The following morning brings another cause for wonderment. Six big Africans enter my room with luggage and packages. They have emptied my room at the hospital.

"But why my private things?"

The Africans are sad and ashamed. One of them explains that the Great Doctor gave the order. But they all like us and do not want us to leave. They follow my preparatory instructions, the first simple steps on the road to health, happiness, and longevity, and they are hopeful of being freed from their present fatal imprisonment. (Their feet and arms are paralyzed or hollowed.)

Sitting among our luggage and packages, we are stranded, left alone.

"Are we now evicted? How brutal and coarse! Turned out to sleep in the jungle!"

To my amazement, Jotsuna does not cry. Her eyes shine with iron will. This is surprising in such a fragile woman, especially deep in the African jungle. She is lighthearted—at least she appears to be.

"The bigger the front," she says, "the bigger the back. Isn't it true? We've suffered the greatest hardships since we left Japan, which can only mean that we must be nearing the greatest joy. This is certain. Look, your body has been devoured, eaten alive, and you are covered with sores. Our luggage has been ransacked. You have been turned out by the Great Doctor, the man you most admired in all the world! Disappointment, total disillusionment—aren't you desperate yet? Haven't you reached your limit?"

Our hardships have lit an inextinguishable fire in Jotsuna, this frail little woman. Strange, isn't it?

Three days later, I cross the garden and climb the sweeping stairway of the minister's big house. Everyone is amazed. Is this the dead man resurrected?

I show the ulcers. No more pus, no more blood. My entire body is dry and smooth.

"You are cured? But this is *unbelievable!* Yes, you told me I'd see a 'miracle,' but *this...*"

A visitor happened to be present, a young hospital doctor who had followed my preparatory instructions very strictly for one week. He had come expressly to see whether I had died yet. Afterwards, knowing he had carried the news to Dr. Schweitzer, I waited a few days, hoping for an invitation to the hospital. But nobody came—neither Miss Emma nor her sick African boy. Nobody.

February 10: I travel with Jotsuna by canoe to the hospital compound. I walk up the beach and the little road leading to the Great

Doctor's house. Many Africans greet us cheerfully.

"Oh, Doctor, you've come back! You will stay with us forever this time, won't you? We've been waiting for you!"

"Are you feeling better?" I ask. "Good. You don't drink too much anymore?"

"Oh no, Doctor, not even a single drop. Look, I feel much, much better. But you will stay with us, won't you? We'll build you a new hospital just like the one here."

"It depends. If the Great Doctor allows me to stay..."

"Bravo!" they shout.

The Great Doctor looks at us in disbelief. He does not touch my feet, which I show him. Nor does he utter a word. However, he carefully examines Jotsuna's hands, which had been afflicted with two or three ulcers. Still, he does not speak. I long to hear the questions, "How have you cured yourself? With what? Can you save all these patients?"

Instead, nonchalantly, he inquires, "When are you leaving?"

"Soon," I answer.

"Would you like to have dinner with us? Can you wait?"

"Thank you very much, but I must go back to the Andende Mission. They are expecting me."

I cannot eat such a costly and luxurious meal while surrounded by millions of poor Africans.

In Andende, I wait patiently for the Great Doctor to see that he was wrong and to invite us back to help him. I wait...one day, two days, three days, five days, ten. Thirteen in all. Nothing...

February 23: With sad hearts, we board the plane for war-torn Algiers to spend a few days in Bougie where my spiritual brother Gabriel, whom I have not seen in sixty-three years, has been expecting me for a long time.

Oh! my simple, self-taught French, learned in Japan, has left me incapable of explaining the practical dialectic, womb of all civilization, all philosophy and all religions, to the greatest pacifist in the world! How sad! My supreme hope has vanished. Shall I be able to find another?

We cross the Sahara in moonlight. I cannot sleep. I think of my brothers and sisters, so poor, so unhappy, who perish daily in the lush green jungle because a magnificent civilization brutally imposes on them its will, its way of thinking and living.

Cancer: Enemy or Benefactor of Mankind?

The last fortress of Oriental civilization, "Invincible Japan," which had strengthened itself through application of the technical and industrial methods of the Occident, was brought to its knees when the first two atomic bombs were dropped in 1945. More than 318,000 civilians in the peaceful cities of Hiroshima and Nagasaki were slaughtered in a few seconds. Moreover, millions of others were poisoned or mutilated, and several thousand more are still dying each year as a consequence of these acts.

Oriental civilization had been moral, as Gandhi's nonviolent strategy demonstrated. But "Invincible Japan," the best student of the Occident, had been attempting to "westernize" itself for eighty years. General Tojo, a simplistic and fanatical military leader, wanted to prove that the student had become superior to the master. What arrogance! He forgot the Oriental teachings he had learned in his youth, especially the strategy of Song Tzu: the strategy of love.

The total defeat of "Invincible Japan" was an event without precedent in our history, as a consequence of which we have voluntarily detached ourselves from the use of military force. "Invincible Japan" no longer exists. Everything changes; everything disappears in this ephemeral, relative world. Nothing remains constant or eternal—except the law of transmutation: Yin-Yang: Change.

Unlike Japan, the United States was victorious. Yet, it suffers other, more serious, difficulties. It has, according to reports, produced 60,000 hydrogen bombs. The Soviet Union possesses 30,000 more. With these 90,000 hydrogen bombs, all of humanity can be annihilated seventy-five times over! Such a situation shatters prospects for lasting peace in a new and frightening way. *Peace through threats is the peace of death.*

In addition to strategic difficulties, the United States confronts biological, physiological, mental, and moral dilemmas: cancer, allergies, diabetes, heart and circulatory diseases, and above all, mental and moral (criminal) illnesses are increasing. Americans now devote $300 per person each year to the cure and prevention of these diseases (this figure does not include money spent by the government or private institutions). The total outlay is $54,000,000,000! Yet the number of sick people increases constantly, and many new diseases continue to appear, the majority of which are directly caused by doctors and medicines—iatrogenic diseases (from the Greek "iatros": doctor and "genesis": origin).

This is why man—and especially "civilized" man—lives in constant uncertainty and fear. The medicine of modern civilization offers no hope for lasting health. This is the way things stand today.

Occidental medicine has clearly made enormous progress. Hardly 150 years have passed since Françoise Quesney liberated surgery from the confines of the barber shop. In these few years, more progress has been made than in the 2300 previous years that separate it from the time of Hippocrates. Undeniably, large hospitals can now be found almost everywhere, and countless others are under construction. But the *number of sick people and of newly discovered diseases is increasing at the same time.* And more: cancer remains invincible! Actually, all the other diseases are *equally* invincible— "cures" are only apparent. Western medicine believes it has succeeded when it has eliminated symptoms or *immediate* consequences; it is not concerned with causes.

But germs or viruses do not cause infectious disease. There are people with natural immunity against *all* such organisms! The question is, rather, *why* do certain individuals lose this natural immunity? And *why* does Western medicine not seek true causes?

Our drastically limited Western vision and the social cancer of rapidly increasing mental illness and crime surely oblige us to think through once more the problems of scientific and technological civilization—particularly the problem of symptomatic medicine, which we so hastily and impulsively adopted nearly a century ago. Let us reconsider that Oriental civilization that was so naively abandoned upon first contact with the brilliant Occidental achievements of technology, power, comfort, and convenience. In many ways, a diametrical opposition existed. The Western will was directed toward satisfaction of sensory and sentimental desires; whereas in the East, the goal was Self-realization. Orientals wished to know the meaning of life, of the world, and of the universe. Seventh Heaven, they believed, could be seen, felt, and known only by moderating desires and overcoming difficulties and sentimental sorrows in this relative world. Then only would they find Absolute Justice (Eternal Happiness and Infinite Liberty) (Oneness).

The Western way is easy; the other is quite difficult. Observing the dangerous precipice to the very edge of which the former way has led mankind, the elderly author of these lines feels profound regret. He calls to mind the sages of the East who lived on this planet thousands of years ago and who still live in their words, which give us hope and courage. They were truly free men: Lao Tzu, Song Tzu, Buddha, Nagarjuna... Is there today enough silence that their message can be heard?

Poor and orphaned at the age of ten, I did not have to suffer through the torments of a modern education during my youth. (All things considered, this was a blessing.) Instead, I worked hard to absorb the traditional teachings that were still alive in the daily life of Japan in those days.

But, I was *extremely* poor and miserable, and this contributed to my eagerness to become acquainted with the benefits of Western civilization. Now, today, I am a rarity: a Japanese of the most traditional type who has lived more than 20 years in the Occident. So it is true, the bigger the front, the bigger the back—the greater the unhappiness, the greater the happiness! Poverty and difficulties alone give us strength to hunger and thirst for justice. In like manner, even if you are suffering from a dread disease such as cancer, if you wish to change, you can do so.

Suffering from pulmonary tuberculosis, I was fortunately abandoned by Western medicine at the age of eighteen. My mother had died of it at 30, my only younger brother at 16, and my little sisters too. My family was one of thousands upon thousands that disappeared because of their inability to adapt to the new, foreign civilization. But, by 20, I had saved myself, thanks to the practice of the teachings of the ancient sages—free men. I owed my survival to the Unifying Principle, mother of all Oriental sciences and techniques.

The teachings of Jesus were simultaneously a systematic medicine, a code of ethics, and an outline of behavior—in short, an authentic, genuine recipe for happiness. Because we are body and soul, better matter and spirit are two aspects of but one existence, we can act on disease by approaching it from either side. Treatment from the material side is necessarily easier, but it is also symptomatic and endless; whereas treatment of the spirit, while more difficult, is basic and fundamental. That is why Jesus saved so many sick and "incurable" people in such apparently miraculous fashion.

The golden method of Jesus is *prayer and fasting*. It is also the basic technique of all Eastern schools that, today as thousands of years ago, direct us toward awareness that we are always in the Kingdom of Eternal Happiness. A master of Buddhism, Taoism, Shintoism, the philosophies of India, or any other traditional religion *is not permitted to fall ill or be killed by assassination or accident under any circumstances*. Whenever I visit Catholic or Protestant hospitals in Europe, the United States, Africa or India, I am severely shocked to see that they all practice the therapeutics of official "scientific" medicine. What a disgrace! What a scandal! They show more confidence in the power of medications and medical treatment than they do in the all-embracing power of the God whose omnipotence they profess to believe in! If a religion cannot guarantee health, the fundamental basis of happiness, then I consider it false: a mere opiate. All the great religions of the Far East promise us immediate happiness in *this* world, not in some "other" world or paradise of wishful thinking. If a religion cannot offer happiness here and now, it is false and deceitful, nothing more than a superstition.

Another way of saying "pray and fast" is "vivere parvo," which means: "Be detached from all that is not absolutely and immediately necessary. Eat and drink only the absolute necessary minimum, remembering that quantity changes quality—and that each individual needs are different."

If this path leads toward Eternal Happiness (awareness of Absolute Justice) as taught by Jesus, Buddha, Lao Tzu, and many others, then is such awareness not within the reach of everyone? Scientific and technological civilization is the nightmare-come-true of man's insane and insatiable greed. In reaction, all traditional sages of the modern Orient are opposed to it: Gandhi, Aurobindo, Tagore, Tensin Okakura, Mao-Tse-Tung, and all present-day non-academic and unofficial great masters of philosophy, morality, and tradition such as M. Taniguchi, S. Yasuoka, and I. Tsuneoka. They would all generally agree with Dr. Francis Magendie, who wrote, "If there were neither doctors nor midwives, man would be in much better health, and much happier." In the West itself, many such as Thoreau, Rousseau, and Edward Carpenter saw the flaws in the Occidental way ("conquer nature").

If Christ were to return to this world of abundance and excess where we eat and drink only to satisfy our desires, he would be astounded. It seems to me that he would begin by immediately abolishing all churches and defrocking all monks who are "as fat as monks." And, if he happened to observe the pedestrians on Fifth Avenue in New York City, he would undoubtedly cry out, "You eat too much! You even eat imported and out-of-season foods. Oh, sons and daughters of vipers! You pray, 'Give us each day our daily bread,' and yet you eat only a token slice accompanied by a thick slab of beef. You gorge yourself on ice cream and tropical fruits, then wash it down with gallons of coffee! Moreover, what you call 'bread' is bleached and sterilized by synthetic chemicals and mechanically kneaded out of lifeless, over-refined flour. Do you want to commit suicide? Do you want to attain Hell at any price, the quicker the better? Are you that ignorant, that arrogant, that mad? Stop! You have forgotten the Order of the Universe and you have violated the order of man. See it clearly: *mea culpa, mea culpa*. My fault!"

The uncertainty, fear, danger, and anguish that reign in present-day civilization—glory of science and technology—are the very ills that plagued King Midas. As you may recall, everything he touched turned to gold, making it impossible for him to eat. Similarly, Western civilization is in control (or seemingly so) of matter. But absolute materialization is total immobilization, *and therefore death*. Life, on the contrary, is infinite mobility, a never-ending transmutation.

Lao-Tzu said, "One produces two; two produces three; and three produces everything." I would like to be his interpreter for you. "One, the Infinite, beginning without beginning, produces two poles—Yin and Yang—eternal antagonists that are strongly attracted to one another because they are antagonistic. Wherever they meet, a desperate struggle ensues and, from this encounter, is born a third antagonist. It is in this manner that all phenomena (visible and invisible) are created. All consequent creations are necessarily more and more complicated and differentiated. This is why our lives are amusing and full of conflicts; some rise and others fall, the first becomes the last, the strongest becomes the weakest, and this perpetual war continues without end. Such is the order of human life in this finite world.

Two poles, Yin and Yang, produce electro-magnetic energy. This energy produces sub-atomic particles, which condense into atoms. These first atoms multiply (multiple isotopes reveal to us the transitions from one type of atom to another). Finally, atoms organize themselves into diverse molecules and these into organisms, according to the universal order of the infinite One. There is no conflict. Everything proceeds smoothly, easily, and naturally. And herein lies the most precious secret: Effortless transmutation can be accomplished through application of the law of Yin and Yang, the Unifying Principle of the philosophy of the Far East. If one applies this Unifying Principle in daily life, there will be very little conflict, difficulty, uncertainty, or fear. Vegetables live peacefully, without speaking or complaining. Animals, too, live amicably most of the time. They admittedly engage in temporary struggles, but they never display any systematic aggressiveness aimed at total destruction of the enemy, slaughter of millions of beings, or sterilization of the planet.

Western civilization contemplates an ideal world in which one can satisfy all sensory desires at will. In the East, on the other hand, one envisions a life of *cooperation with nature and with one's fellow man*. Religion, philosophy, and myriad art forms are the flowers of Oriental culture; whereas force, technology, and world dominion are the flowers of Western civilization (whose blossom is the hydrogen bomb).

In the past 100 years, it is true, Orientals, and particularly the Japanese, have abandoned and forgotten this Unifying Principle. Nowadays, in Japan, no official institutions for its promulgation exist, whereas formerly all schools taught it, for thousands of years. Life itself was considered an omni-present classroom in which one could learn the Unifying Principle and the Order of the Universe.

The Chinese ideogram (文明), which designates Western civilization, is erroneous: "the world enlightened by the lamp of philosophy (i.e., the Unifying Principle that shows us that all antagonisms are complementary)." Perhaps their insight into the future was very clear. But, as things stand now, the West should rather be represented by characters that signify "the world burnt by the torch of technology (i.e., materialism, dualism, and atheism)."

Fear of viruses, cancer, mental disease, crime, invasion—fear is the hallmark of the scientific and technical Western civilization. But can this civilization continue to accuse others, outsiders, of being responsible, with claims of infestation by "Asian flue" or "Communist plots"? The ills of society and the individual are not products of the external environment. The Western world itself has created them, cancer included. Cancer is autogenous, self-produced. But the Westerner is incapable of perceiving his errors. Why? Because these errors are too large! And what are they? *Dualisms*—analytical and mechanical dualisms. Materialistic, egocentric dualisms!

Since the time of Aristotle, and especially since the time of

Descartes, non-material problems have been brushed aside. Western man has concerned himself only with matter, more and more forgetting non-matter, even to the point of utterly denying its existence! He has come to believe that all problems can be solved through analytical identification of their various component parts. But chemistry and physics have discovered that chemical molecules are not the final components of this world; that atoms are not either, despite Democratus's ancient definition; and, in fact, that atoms and the sub-atomic particles from which they are formed derive from energy sources *whose origin is absolutely unknown!* All scientific research has been thrown into confusion by this last discovery. Professor P.W. Bridgman, for example, committed suicide at the age of 79 when his "orderly" idea of the cosmos was shattered by this discovery.

Occidental medicine, which has fumblingly advanced by clinging to the principles of physics and chemistry, is completely helpless before the increasing numbers of "incurable" diseases: cancer, allergies, mental illness, heart ailments, and so on. Modern Western medicine has believed that the fundamental basis of life can be found at the chemical level, that is, at the level of the external electron layer of the atom. But the true picture is far different! The roots of life go much deeper, to the level of the nuclei and further. Modern experts are seeking the vital mechanism in electromagnetic resonance, electronic spin, in natural and biological transmutation. But, even if they could conjure up a correct image of the ultra-infinitesimal structure of matter, they would never be able to determine the nature of what animates it; namely, the invisible: Life itself.

History shows us that, invariably, all great empires and civilizations began to decay from within. The responsibility for such deterioration must rest with the leadership, king or government, whose idea of the natural order of things leads the people. A faith and a will that are securely based on an accurate concept of life, the world and the universe are therefore necessary.

For more than ten years, we have been approaching a crisis that is extraordinary and without precedent in the history of man. Western civilization has advanced too rapidly, too materialistically. Will it pause to reflect on the origin of its uncertainty, its fear that war might erupt at any moment, its suspicion that the whole of humanity is being devoured by cancer?

Cancer is autogenous. *If it were caused by a virus, how could people in good health resist it so easily?* Admitting the existence of "natural immunity," we are still left with the problem of explaining that immunity. Yet nothing is known about it. Many Western doctors have declared that cancer is caused by a virus, but no one knows the nature of this hypothetical virus, where it comes from, or how cancer is produced by it. Off on an opposite tack, the United States government identified cigarettes as being responsible for lung-cancer, a conclusion that is based on *statistics alone*. These statistics do not take into consideration the *eating habits* of the subjects.

Yet statistical or virological medicine can accuse just about anyone or anything of being the culprit.

Generally speaking, Westernized Japanese doctors do not accept the virus theory. To my knowledge, only Dr. K. Hasumi has declared himself in its favor. All others attach major significance to the idea of repeated stimulation. This was the most respected explanation of the nineteenth century.

But what *is* cancer?

Cancer does not grow old; it does not fall ill; it develops, stops, sleeps, awakens, and resumes its activities. It repeats such cycles indefinitely. It resists, adapts, triumphs. It is life itself! It is blind, mechanical will, that is to say insatiability, voracity, uncontrolled growth. It is, therefore, unbalanced. Too much of the material and not enough of the non-material. Why this disharmony between matter and spirit? Everything has a cause.

The cause of cancer is dualistic, materialistic man. He is like King Midas who, in realizing his most cherished dream, changed everything into gold. Modern Midas attempts to organize the world toward satisfaction of his blind and sensory desires, and the result is cancer, which grows blindly and indefinitely, responsive to the destructive touch of a humanity that has abandoned its soul in favor of the Cartesian or Aristotelian dichotomy. Quantity changes quality. King Midas has lost his perspective and with it his bearings! He no longer perceives, can no longer find meaning in super-abundant matter. Rather he has found the opposite: uncertainty, fear, anguish, war and burgeoning cancer.

Now, he must listen, if he can still hear. Let him only acknowledge the voice of the non-materialistic, metaphysical, moral civilization that lives in cooperation with nature by consciously applying the principles and theorems of the Order of the Universe and the Unifying Principle, and his perspective will return once more. Modern King Midas will rediscover a true paradise in which he is all-powerful, respected by Dionysus, god of wine and pleasure, befriended by Silenus, master of Dionysus, and perfectly free to enjoy the fruits of the garden through which flows the Pactolus with its gold-dust grains. Above all, at his side will be his daughter Marigol, the most beautiful and virtuous girl in the world.

First though, Modern Midas must shed his donkey ears that still prefer the music of Pan's pipe (symbol of the mundane) to that of Apollo's lyre (representing the music of the Seven Heavens). Otherwise, the reeds will keep repeating in the slightest breeze, "Midas, King Midas has donkey ears!" Otherwise, Western technological civilization will never penetrate to the meaning of the Order of the Infinite Universe.

A Thousand and One Ways to Cure Cancer

There are "a thousand and one ways" to cure cancer, using the philosophical-medical approach of the Far East. The same holds true for all other so-called "incurable" diseases.

The Unifying Principle is the practical, paradoxical dialectic expressed in the two words Yin and Yang, which shows that all antagonisms are complementary and permits the transmutation of unhappiness into happiness, difficulty into ease, uselessness into usefulness, hostility into friendship, sickness into health, sadness into joy—not by a psychological turnabout after the manner of William James, but by logical, biological, and physiological means.

"Absurd! Preposterous! A fairy tale!" Such would be the comments of Valery and Bergson.

But, after all, is not our life itself a fairy tale? Do we not inhabit a world of miracles, as did Alice in Wonderland? Do we not travel through infinite space on a gigantic sphere rotating at the enormous speed of 1,000 miles an hour? And yet we are not catapulted into space! Is it not miraculous? What keeps us from falling off, according to Newton, is a "universal force of attraction." But what is the universal force? *No one has ever explained it!* It is a mere hypothesis. Moreover, according to present theory, this tremendous force is *non-existent in the nuclear realm,* which is the fundamental basis of our own existence. And that definitely complicates things. For, if this force does not exist at the fundamental level of our existence, how can it still be called universal?

Unnoticed by the West and nearly forgotten by Orientals themselves, the philosophy of the Far East opens up horizons quite different from those of science and technology. Included are marvels such as the Flying Carpet and Aladdin's Lamp. Missing in the wondrous world of this philosophy are sickness (especially of the "incurable" variety), inhumane war, and crime. Uncertainty, fear, and cancer are replaced by light, joy, and gratitude toward everyone and everything forever!

In reality, the difference between East and West is much more profound than is generally suspected. Since I have been acquainted with Europe for more than fifty years, I am particularly aware of this. In certain ways, I feel like a complete stranger in the Occident, although generally it has been quite pleasant to be here. Something seems to be missing. This civilization is too mechanical, too artificial, too smart, too solid, too rigid, too symmetrical and geometric—altogether too perfect, brilliant, inhumane, and cold. It is lacking in fairy tales!

*Shibu, wabi, and sabi** are unknown in the West. Essential and fundamental to our way of life, they are difficult for civilized people to appreciate. The ambassador-poet Paul Claudel, who loved Japan and its art, admitted that he could not understand them, not even intellectually.

The difference between East and West is not only a matter of mentality. The rift, in fact, goes much deeper—to basic ways of looking at the universe. The difference is as that between reality and a photograph—the one alive and the other dead. The Orient is much more sentimental, indefinite, indirect and intangible, yet much more profound; its people are more modest, reserved, and engaging; while Westerners are by contrast more talkative, proud, and vain. The former is like a new-born baby, fresh with vitality itself; the latter is like

*Shibu means "modest elegance" (as opposed to "glamour"). Wabi means "complete aloneness" (as opposed to being a "club member"). Sabi means "quality of being aged or worn by nature" (as opposed to "shiny brand-newness"). (These are all approximations, as they are very difficult or impossible to translate.)

a middle-aged woman who knows her way around.

The civilization of the East is poetic—that of the West is prosaic. Poetry and aesthetics are missing in the Occident: *wabi, sabi, and shibu.*

The East is a land of fairy-tales, a world of "a thousand and one nights," childlike and amusing. We prefer it to a society steeped in uncertainty and fear. If you were to visit us sometime, we are entirely at your disposal.

*   *   *

The birthplace of Buddhism was India. A few centuries after the death of Buddha, Buddhism separated into two quite distinct sects: Hinayana and Mahayana. The latter is the Great Vehicle or Big Door, the wide-open way, large, paradoxical, free, philosophical, and cosmogonical (pertaining to the origin of the universe). The former is the Small Vehicle or Little Door, the limited way, scrupulous, ordinary, rich in cults and rites. Neither exists in India any longer! Both have been exported, Hinayana to the south and Mahayana to the north.

Mahayana crossed Asia, took root in China, and proceeded to Japan, where it is very much alive today. In fact, most of the philosophy and medicine of Indian origin has undergone change in the crossing of Asia.

The word "philosophy" in the Orient is not at all the same as in the Occident. To a Westerner, philosophy means an accumulation of physical, technical, and metaphysical knowledge, and therefore something *relative*. To his Eastern brother, however, philosophy means a study of the Order that gives birth to and governs everything in this universe and all universes and is, therefore, transcendental, *absolute*. Occidental philosophy is dependent upon (or at least influenced by) physical and technical knowledge, resulting in today's nuclear sciences that are lost in an infinitesimal, microscopic world: an impasse. Oriental philosophy, on the other hand, is panoramic, *independent of physical knowledge,* and seeks understanding of the ruling principles of the universe. Western physical sciences, based on dualism, divide and subdivide indefinitely, while in the Orient all sciences and philosophies are dialectically unified.

Oriental medicine is only one application of the dialectic philosophy, which considers every antagonism as complementary. Because the Infinite Universe is the source of all phenomena, both health and sickness are, therefore, manifestations of the Order of the Universe. An illness and its symptoms are not *violations* of the Order of the Universe, but are rather evidence of *a lack of understanding* of the Order of the Universe. Therefore, the cure must be educative, rather than remedial or symptomatic. Such educative medicine, necessarily philosophical, was the foundation of the approach of Jesus. It is very understandable to Orientals that he was generally successful, in spite of the questionability of certain specific "miracles" in the Christian gospels. For this reason, the cases of healing reported in the Bible are worthy of study by scientific minds.

Claude Bernard, one of the greatest modern Occidental scientists, gave us some very sensible advice in his *Introduction to the Study of Experimental Medicine:*

> In the field of science, no opinion has absolute authority.
>
> One must not wish to defend his opinion at all costs.
>
> The most important rule for the scientist is always to be ready to change his views, to develop and enlarge his thought.
>
> Truths in the experimental sciences being relative, science can only advance through revolution and absorption of ancient truths in a new scientific form.
>
> There is no room for personal authority in the experimental sciences. Such authority impedes that progress of science.
>
> Unknowing reverence for personal authority in the experimental sciences would be a superstition and would constitute a real obstacle to all progress.
>
> Great men are precisely those who have brought forth new ideas and swept away error.

If you are a scientist after the manner of Claude Bernard, you will surely delight in visiting the wonderland where so-called sickness is non-existent. There, butterflies dance all day long with the joy of living, and insects chant of love the night through. Neither doctors nor hospitals flourish. All sickness is healed automatically. No such thing as a "miraculous" cure is admitted. In fact, if there *were* "incurable" diseases that did not heal spontaneously, *that* would the "miracle!"

But the inhabitants of this wonderland, being very childlike, curious, and amicable, have over the past 100 years imported the whole of Occidental civilization. It has cost them dearly: thousands upon thousands of families have perished. Expecting help from the new medicine that had replaced their ancient, traditional one, they experience increasingly disastrous results. The more they applied the new medicine, the more they suffered. The more quickly large hospitals were erected, the more new patients came to fill them. And, as the pharmaceutical industry prospered, so did the number of invalids and corpses increase.

Having relentlessly studied and practiced the new medicine, the intellectuals and the rich of Japan have come closer and closer to the point of completely rejecting it. Many have returned to the traditional way (which is no longer legally or officially approved). In ever-growing numbers, they resort to moxa, acupuncture, and ancient Chinese techniques. And "miraculous" cures occur! The superiority of traditional medicine is being experimentally rediscovered after a lapse of several decades. Astonishingly, many precious treasures have been recovered, not the least of which is the source of this "miraculous" medicine, the dialectical philosophy of Yin and Yang—glory of Oriental civilization and fundamental basis of the great religions of man. Here we can learn *how* to find Infinite Liberty, Eternal Happiness, and Absolute Justice.

The renaissance of ancient Japan has begun with a reevaluation of the national tradition that over a period of more than a thousand years, developed from the civilizations of India and China. Today, many Japanese are reinvestigating this mother-philosophy of all sciences, cultures, and techniques and, with deep gratitude, are delving into the works of ancient, long-forgotten masters, through whom tradition still lives.

But these great masters are *totally unknown* in the West! Although they represent the soul of the Eastern peoples, they are unintelligible to the civilized scientists and technologists of the modern West. I have made many efforts, living in the West for decades, to make available a simplified and comprehensively scientific form of the Unifying Principle, but have everywhere encountered nearly impenetrable misunderstanding. Orientals have imported all of Western civilization with facility and pleasure, since Western civilization is visible, materialistic, technical, and easily imitable. But Oriental civilization, being philosophical, spiritual, and invisible, escapes the grasp of the civilized. It is, however, *essential* the East and West understand one another.

If such understanding is to develop, each party must first forsake its arrogance. This can require a high price: utter failure, or even loss of life or sanity. The timeless command, "Know thyself," cannot be carried out through a pat formula. We must realize that, according to application of Oriental philosophy, *"ego" or "self" is a combination of ignorance and arrogance*. Masters of Eastern philosophy know this and, therefore, remain silent. Shunning publicity or self-advertisement, they live humbly with their students.

As a consequence, foreign visitors encounter great difficulties when trying to find them, and those with any reputation at all are to one degree or another Europeanized or Americanized. The real masters conceal themselves, often deep in the mountains.

In this, my seventy-first year on this planet, I decided to spend several months in Japan for the first time in twelve years. One evening, I invited a few traditionalist Japanese to study with me what we should do in the face of the uncertainties and fears that rule the civilized world. Here is a partial guest list:

T. Katayama,	76, ex-prime minister
Dr. K. Takahashi,	90, founder and director for over 50 years of the largest ear and nose hospital in Japan

Dr. K. Hutaki,	90, Honorary President of the Shuyodan, the oldest moral and traditional movement
M. Hasunuma,	82, Director of the Shuyodan
T. Nishida,	93, leader of the *Ittoen* movement, the oldest religious group for public services
I. Tsuneoka,	65, ex-senator, President of the Central Institute
Mme. R. Hiratsuka,	78, President of the Confederation of Japanese Feminist Societies
M. Taniguchi,	72, Founder-President of the *Seicho House*, the largest modern religious and moral organization in Japan
S. Yasuoka,	65, President of *Siyuhkai*, one of the most powerful philosophical and moral groups
M. Nakano,	45, Secretary General of the International Cultural Organization

All of these traditionalist Japanese personalities answered my call. We discussed conditions at length and decided to open an information center covering all cultural, moral, and philosophical movements for the benefit of those who wish to study Oriental philosophy as an integral part of the daily life of traditional Japanese. First on the agenda will be to teach how to cure so-called "incurable" illness (cancer, allergies, diabetes, heart and mental diseases, etc.) through application of the Unifying Principle.

The book you are now reading was conceived as an introduction to this international movement.

It was also decided to make available a list of "incurable" diseases that *had* been cured, especially cancer, describing the patient's age, sex, history, and biological and physiological recovery. There is, of course, insufficient room for such a list here, but to all interested parties, complete information is readily accessible. Moreover, on-the-spot examination of actual cases can be provided for those who are able to visit Japan in person.

One of the aims of this little book will be achieved if it succeeds in introducing to the West the general principles of Eastern philosophy-medicine, a way of life that is capable of curing every one of the illnesses declared "incurable" by Occidental medicine.

Dear civilized friends, this medicine-philosophy may still seem unintelligible to you. Please be patient and remember that the theories of Copernicus, Galileo, and Einstein were also initially considered incomprehensible. Most importantly, do not confuse modernized, technical, industrial Japan, imitator of the civilized world, with its traditional ancestor. Spiritual and invisible, the latter is in hiding and seldom appears in public. But, if you wish to learn more about it, read the works of Lafcadio Hearn (1850-1905) who, as a young reporter, had the great good fortune of discovering humanity's masterpiece: the Japanese woman!

I can also recommend *Zen in the Art of Archery* by Professor Eugen Herrigel, a pistol champion who abandoned his "killer-sidearm" in favor of the Japanese bow. His six year stay in Japan provided him with profound understanding of himself through application of the principles of Zen, whose basis is the Unifying Principle of Yin and Yang.

Miracles

There exist in Japan more than fifteen distinct schools concerned with the subjects of religion, ethics, culture, and physical science. Some teach how to lead a healthy life through study of tradition or practice of various forms of religious worship. Others teach simple and practical symptomatic techniques for the healing of any sickness. These latter are not so concerned as the former with the larger, more difficult problems of familial and societal disruption.

Basically the schools can be divided as follows:

1. Cultural School
2. Philosophical School (studying works of ancient sages of China and Japan)
3. Shinto School
4. Buddhist School
5. Spiritualist School
6. Psychic School
7. Fakir School
8. School of Yoga
9. School of Ayurveda
10. School of the Medicine of Jesus (not to be confused with what Americans call "Christian Science")
11. School of Acupuncture and Moxa (symptomatic treatment)
12. School of Chinese Medicine
13. School of Massage (symptomatic treatment)
14. School of Palm Healing (symptomatic treatment)
15. School of Macrobiotics (nutritional)
16. Various other schools of modern symptomatic treatments

Several hundred thousand Japanese belong to these schools, whose "healers" exceed by two to three times the number of "Westernized" doctors. And although the number of student-disciples is probably ten times greater than those who subscribe to Western methods, *General MacArthur ordered the complete abandonment of all such practices and disciplines during his occupation of Japan.* It appears that soon these ancient arts may be utterly lost.

Most of those who come to learn from traditional healers are former patients who were abandoned by "official medicine" or who grew tired of uselessly spending money to secure ineffective care. Among them are many who had reached the point of desperation, their cases considered terminal and their consequent cures, therefore, "miraculous."

Mr. M. Taniguchi, founder-president of *Seicho House* (house of life), is one of Japan's most esteemed experts in Oriental philosophy. His followers number in the millions, and he has published more than one hundred books. Editor of several monthly newspapers for more than thirty years, he owns his own press and publishing house and is director of a university-size school in Tokyo.

The teaching of Taniguchi has saved countless condemned "incurables," including cancer victims. His method is ethical and philosophical—in no way symptomatic. He teaches that everyone is born free, happy, and wise, and that if one fails, the cause lies within oneself. It is his conviction that in order to restore his health, man needs only to establish by himself and for himself his own freedom *through reflection on his origin, i.e., his nature as a son of God, of the Infinite-Absolute-One.*

Are there not as many spontaneous and miraculous cures in the West? Of course. But "scientific" doctors refuse to acknowledge the existence of these "miraculous" cures because they do not yet understand their mechanism! They are interested only in cases that admit of microscopic analysis or quantitative measurement. However, in his book, *Cancer*, Dr. W. Nakahara, President of the Cancer Center of Japan, cites several interesting cases:

1. Dr. L. Stuart, Chief of Pathology at Memorial Hospital of

New York, who enjoys an outstanding reputation stemming from his more than thirty years of practice as a cancer specialist, operated on a woman suffering from cancer of the uterus in 1946. The case was desperate, and the woman was abandoned. Six years later, however, this same woman happened to be examined once again by Dr. Stuart and to his amazement was found to be completely free of cancer!

2. In the same hospital, which is located in the Jewish section of New York, one-third of the female cancer patients are Jewish. In the last ten years, death due to cancer in these patients has been limited to 26 out of 702 cases, producing only a 3.7% mortality rate! In other words, more than 96% of these Jewish women have cured themselves spontaneously! Is this not remarkable?

"Miracles" exist everywhere—or rather, miracles exist in the minds of the ignorant, those who refuse to see through the superficial shell of appearance, among whom are many practitioners of "scientific" medicine.

3. In issue 13 of *Planète*, a Parisian monthly magazine, a feature by Roger Wybott entitled "A Different Medicine: Acupuncture" provides accurate information concerning the life and works of a Frenchman named Soulié de Morant who, while still quite young, spent twenty years in China as French Consul General. After retiring, he labored to introduce acupuncture to Europe. I met him for the first time in 1930 and helped him in my capacity as a practitioner of acupuncture, giving him more than 2,000 pages of informative documents. Unfortunately, when I returned to Europe in 1956 after a 23-year absence, he had died.

Soulié de Morant dedicated thirty years of his life to introducing a foreign medical technique that is now officially practiced in all French national hospitals. More than 5,000 licensed physicians are utilizing it in France and Germany, and for the past twelve years, the Parisian newspapers have been giving it frequent and thorough coverage.

Also interesting is the note concerning Roger Wybott, author of this article, which appeared in a forward:

The name Roger Wybott may surprise you. He was Chief of Staff of the Territories from the end of the war until 1958. In 1948, he was suffering from stomach complications. He had tried, in vain, all manner of treatments. His case was inoperable. Fortunately, he met Soulié de Morant, and their first acupuncture session cured him completely. Since then, he has been doing his best to propagate this practical, provocative, and extremely effective medicine. His latest book, *Culturel Fluids*, has just been published.

There are thousands of "miraculous cures" every day, not only in the Orient but also in the West. Doctors and professors of medicine, however, have scant time to study them, being inundated with reports of new surgical techniques and chemical products designed to counteract the ever-widening spectrum of symptoms. One should remember that their operational funds for medical research come for the most part from the pharmaceutical industry.

4. An intriguing story entitled "Are We Well-Cared-For?" appeared in issue 169 (Feb. 1960) of *Realités* Magazine:

Miss V. P., raised in Morocco, had a very delicate stomach. At the age of 25, following an evening in which she had drunk three cocktails, she experienced sharp abdominal pains. These "spasms" or "grips" were accompanied by vomiting, colic, and fever. Her doctor methodically checked for typhoid fever, amoebic dysentery, and collibacillosis. His final diagnosis was "colitis," for which he prescribed intestinal disinfectants, bismuth, and a simple diet. Slowly, Miss P. recovered.

From time to time over the following years, the attacks recurred whenever she strayed from her diet so that eventually, at the age of 35, she was compelled to maintain a regimen she considered austere: broiled meat, cooked vegetables, no fruits, nothing raw, no alcohol, no milk, no seafood, and no sauces. She complained, "I'm obliged to eat like an old woman." But spontaneous recovery occurred as if from some unknown cause.

As has been said, certainly neither East nor West lacks "miracles." It remains for true scientists, such as Claude Bernard, to investigate these cases.

Yet, in the annals of official medicine, the number of "incurables" is fantastically high. Many patients follow useless, hopeless trails for years. Many others discard official medicine in despair and, if wealthy enough, haunt the emporiums of quacks and charlatans; or take to their beds, awaiting the end with a feeling of loneliness, "abandoned by man and God." In addition, the mentally ill greatly outnumber the physically stricken. In spite of the great strides of modern medicine, there are many more forsaken and hopeless patients in the West than in the East.

I know a Parisian woman doctor who owns a luxurious apartment in the heart of the city that is complete with physical-culture studio, lecture room, and clinic. She represents French official medicine at various international congresses and lectures in universities and hospitals. But when I met her, she had been suffering from an "incurable" bladder ailment for more than twenty years! Of course, she had tried all available symptomatic treatments, but in vain.

Imagine: a famous doctor who cannot cure herself in twenty years! Incredible!

My wife and I were invited to live with her to see what we could do to assist her. After only ten days of Jotsuna's macrobiotic cuisine, *she was completely cured*. For the first time in 23 years, not one microbe in her urine!

This woman doctor owned two villas, one near Paris and the other in the south of France. She was very kind and invited us to stay as long as we wished. But we left the moment she was cured, for she refused to study the philosophy of our medicine. Perhaps she was too set in her ways.

I remember very well a day on which she introduced a few of her patients to me. The first was a gentleman of about 45 whom she said she had been treating for 17 years, adding, "He's so weak he needs treatments once or twice a month." Unbelievable—17 years with the same illness! It was the same with the second patient, the third, the fourth—all were "old" patients.

I was shocked. According to our philosophy of medicine, it is unthinkable that a master should fall ill except for a common cold every ten years or so. It is equally unimaginable that he should be unequipped to cure himself of *anything*, even a wart. For how could a master who publicly teaches methods of healing and of keeping fit fall ill himself? What a fraud! What a swindle! In Japan, such a charlatan would have to execute his own justice: harakiri!

Almost the entire population over forty in the United States and France suffers from one or more chronic illnesses. Hospitals flourish like mushrooms after rainfall, clearly indicating the sickness of the nations—indeed, of civilization itself. How many like that forty-five-year-old gentleman suffer seventeen years of grueling treatment?

Yet, according to official medicine, each person's red blood cells are completely changed every 10 days through their destruction and replacement at the rate of 2,000 per second. (Ed. note: Recent studies seem to indicate that this occurs in about 3 months.) Even bone cells are renewed in a few months. Why, then, could we not heal or at least greatly improve a patient's condition in ten days (or at most three or four months) by altering the composition of his blood through change of diet? This is what I have been practicing for fifty years. And the "miraculous" cures I have effected are simply physiological, biological, bio-chemical facts.

Nor are my results isolated. Many others have been brought about by master philosophers of the Orient, and many more have occurred spontaneously. Meanwhile, the number of "incurables" increases daily. A recent issue of "The New York Herald Tribune" contained an extensive list of such hopeless and chronic illnesses: allergies, heart and circulatory diseases, cancer, etc. Those suffering from one single allergy alone (hay fever) number 30,000,000 in the United States! In recognition of the needs of the hour, a national congress of U.S. medical specialists declared after long deliberations in 1961 that a "divine" medicine should be concocted, one that would supplant current methods. I should like to suggest a ten-day trial, at the very minimum, of the Oriental philosophy-medicine that I have been demonstrating for many years, and that can cure the millions upon millions of mentally ill, and society itself with its modern artless wars that are only a symptom of the collective moral sickness of mankind.

Let us catch a glimpse of another world, a world of wonder. Let us consider the fish of the ocean which neither age nor fall ill, never know uncertainty or the fear of hydrogen bombs. Let us observe butterflies, insects, and animals that never need doctors, hospitals, or drugstores. Their secret, the secret of living in co-operation with nature, must be made known to Western physicians so that their treatment of the whole wretchedly suffering population of this planet may be improved. We must do away with the arrogance and irresponsibility in modern medical practice that have resulted in more deaths than wars can account for. We must have no more of Dr. Schweitzer, who insists on the importance of life at one moment and then goes on to kill billions of micro-organisms at the next. We must cease this mindless hurling of weaponry on symptoms.

Instead, let us think deeply. What is life, where does it come from, where is it going?

All can be accomplished while loving one's neighbors and even one's "enemies." The microbe can be our benefactor by teaching us how we have erred. Our real need in these times is for a practical, logical philosophy of love that can be applied effectively to everyday life. The "divine" medicine we seek is the medicine of love.

Symptomatic Medicine and Fundamental Medicine

In 1849, Claude Bernard said to his students, "Gentlemen, the scientific medicine I am about to teach you does not exist."

In this finite, limited, relative world, there are two antagonists at all levels: Yin and Yang (centrifugality and centripetality), female and male, woman and man, cold and hot, darkness and light, death and life, sadness and joy, hatred and love, spiritual and material, weak and strong, back and front. Man becomes a dualist when he observes these two sides to phenomena *without seeing their unity*. Antagonism is found at each of our relative levels of judgment: blind, sensory, sentimental, intellectual, social, and philosophical. In reality, these antagonisms are the "heads" and "tails" of the same coin. Extremes of antagonism "touch" each other and commingle. *One kills his lover at the extreme of love!* While this appears contradictory, it is just such contradictions that animate the world and from which man struggles at all cost to save himself. Most men end their lives still puzzled by the enigmas of existence.

Consider, for example, wealth and fame. For years and years, men desperately seek them. Finally succeeding, they awake one day to find their dreams shattered. They have become slaves of their own wealth, are threatened with assassination, attacked because of high reputation, or victimized by a jealousy their own success has aroused.

To understand and *enjoy* such contradiction, one must unveil the Supreme Judgment. This is the explicit purpose of Oriental philoso-

54

phy with its concept of polarizable monism. Strangely enough, this philosophy of dialectical logic has been totally ignored by most of the Western world for nearly 2,000 years—in spite of the fact that *the Celtic civilization was based on it.* Modern civilization, which has colonized nearly all the world, is based on formal logic: relative, conceptual, and materialistic. All exclusive, and therefore alienated, mentalities belong to this group, seldom if ever freeing themselves to grasp the concept of monism. All who see or believe in only *one side* of the coin (good or evil, body or soul, sentimental or intellectual) are dualistic, exclusive, and quarrelsome. Only those who see that the two sides of all phenomena, visible and invisible, are front and back or beginning and end of *One Reality* can embrace any antagonistic situation, see its complementarity, and help others to do the same, thereby establishing peace and harmony. All who are quarrelsome, all who find *anything* intolerable in this world, are dualists. And as long as they remain so, they will never know peace.

Peace cannot be obtained on a collective basis. It is not dependent on others. It is individual and personal and is another name for Perfect Health, Eternal Happiness, and Absolute Freedom, all of which are identical and may be further described as the ability to change sickness to health (and vice versa), unhappiness to happiness (vice versa), and slavery to freedom (and vice versa). He who cannot do so does not know absolute peace. And as long as he continues to live in such schizophrenic isolation from his true identity, he will inevitably die in uncertainty and fear—even in the shelter of an armored fortress defended by 90,000 hydrogen bombs.

And then, there is—*cancer*.

Civilized people consider this disease (a natural phenomenon) as the most terrible curse to which human society has ever been subjected. Such a fear-crazed attitude is exclusive, lonely, and egocentric, signifying a closed mind and a rigid body, and resembles the behavior of a little cat, his back humped and his hair erect before a vicious dog. Such fear (the front) and hostility (the back) become greater and greater and are eventually transformed into aggressive action. Mobilizing all the physical and intellectual means at his dis-

posal (both moral and immoral) in order to destroy his dreaded enemy, cancer, man risks no less than his own simultaneous destruction,
because his cancer and his body are nourished at the same source.
They are Siamese twins sharing the same heart.

Non-civilized people who study and apply the dialectical monistic philosophy are also surprised at the appearance of cancer. But,
they feel neither fear nor hostility. Instead, they react as would a
cheerful, smiling, innocent child who has given him so much to be
thankful for. He is sorry to have caused so much trouble. Such is
the response of non-civilized people toward their universal father,
Tao: the Order of the Infinite Universe. When scolded with cancer,
they examine themselves very deeply in order to discover what they
have done to deserve this reprimand. They understand that nothing
unpleasant or sorrowful is needlessly produced, but that, on the contrary, all is given that is necessary, useful, or agreeable: food, drink,
sun, moon, stars, mountains, fresh air, water, fish, flowers, the atoms,
infinite space, and time. All this is given freely. How can we not accept all with the deepest gratitude? What fools we are to protest.

There is no day without night. Good weather is only appreci-
ated in contrast with bad. The cold of winter is indispensable to the
germination of plant life. Nothing has been needless or destructive
since the beginningless beginning, but has assisted over billions of
years in the embellishment of this planet where we live today so
happily. We have everything we need. Above all, we have life, that
miracle whose structure and function we do not as yet comprehend.
We are puzzled by the nature of memory, which allows us to think
and judge. We wonder over the mechanism that enables us to express
and convey our thoughts in the form of action. We have scant understanding of understanding itself.

Non-civilized people maintain full confidence in the Order of
the Infinite Universe, which is their creator and their source of Absolute Justice. They feel no need to protest. If something occurs which
they find initially more or less difficult to accept, they need only
reflect and study in order to determine the true meaning of the situation. They meditate, forgetting to eat, drink, or even sleep. Night

and day they review events in terms of Yin and Yang. Detached from everything, from abundance and abuse, Supreme Judgment reveals itself, glittering like the sun through a rift in the clouds.

One morning, they awaken and are again happy, joyful, and courageous. They are as active as newborn children, and as equally free of disease. They have cured themselves, as anyone can—even of so-called "hereditary" diseases, which are only the hypothetical concoctions of incapable doctors who are incapable of explaining their actual mechanism (and also, often, of curing them). When we find a disease's cause, we can always cure it. The idea of "hereditary disease" is indicative of a pessimistic view of life according to which we cannot change sickness into health.

When one is detached from everything, especially from eating, one is detached from all diseases, because one is what one eats.

Our civilization, one of abundance and abuse, approves of eating large amounts of food. A particular theory of nutrition that dates back hardly a hundred years recommends that we eat not only thousands of calories but also consume a certain percentage of animal protein each day. Yet, in Asia, hundreds of millions of non-civilized people have lived successfully as vegetarians for *thousands* of years.

Man is free. He can eat defeated, weak, innocent, defenseless beings. Perhaps the latter were born to feed the strong, as the militants of "survival of the fittest" affirm. Well, to each his own—a man's menu can be as varied as his whims.

But, I would like to give you some advice. It is the conclusion I have reached after fifty years of studying and teaching the Unifying Principle of the philosophy of the Far East. In my opinion, it is the key to awareness of the fact that we are always in the Kingdom of Heaven. It can enable you to immunize yourself your entire life against any disease—cancer and mental illness included. The secret is quite simple: avoid animal protein as much as possible and completely avoid refined sugar.

Refined sugar and excess animal protein are the two main causes of all our misfortunes!

You may enjoy animal protein in small quantities. But do not forget that, in accordance with the teachings of the ancient sages, billions of Asians lived well and avoided animal protein for many thousands of years in China and India. One can live without meat and fish. Neither is necessary. But, I repeat, you may eat them for the sake of pleasure. However, restrict your intake if you wish to preserve your physical and mental health. Learn how to *moderate* your animal and sensorial desires.

After studying and teaching traditional Oriental medicine and philosophy for fifty years, and having observed how this "forbidden" medicine has cured thousands of desperate, abandoned, "incurable" patients, I have learned the secret of health and a magnificent life. Here, from my experience, is a list of important suggestions:

1. Suppress sugar completely from your diet.

2. Learn that it is possible to live without being carnivorous.

3. Eat primarily whole grain cereals, vegetables, beans and seaweeds—all as unrefined as possible.

4. Eat as little as possible of other foods (vivere parvo).

5. Keep liquid down to a minimum.

Follow these instructions for one, two, or three weeks. You will see the results for yourself.

Before leaving this subject, I would like to add that industrialized, commercial sugar is totally unnecessary, man having lived without it for *thousands* of years. It exists only for pleasure; and pleasure, being ruled by our lower sensorial judgment, often lures us into great dangers.

Some people find meat delicious. Our civilization of abundance and abuse supplies us with much of it, and the nutritional theory in favor nowadays strongly recommends it. But, in point of fact, meat and other animal proteins are not at all "absolutely necessary." One can live without them. All animals can produce proteins peculiar to their species, even when they lack a source of nitrogen—organic or inorganic. All are endowed with the ability to transmute carbon and oxygen into nitrogen. (See *Biological Transmutations* by Louis Kervran, 1962, Maloine, Paris.)

If, in accordance with modern nutritional theories, we consume large amounts of animal protein, we lose the ability to produce for ourselves our own special proteins. This is a net loss of adaptability—in other words, a decrease in vitality and independence. (The same holds true for insulin and Vitamin C. [Ed. note: The appendix on Vitamin C, which appeared in the original French edition of this book, has been deleted owing to its availability as a *macroguide* from the George Ohsawa Macrobiotic Foundation.] An excess of Vitamin C, moreover, can cause cancer.) In actuality, proteins are produced by the body with excess materials that might be otherwise useless, appearing in storage-form as rapidly growing nails, warts, or skin, especially on the sole of the foot. Cancer is the storage of excess that explodes, and we will examine this phenomenon more deeply later on. But, for now, let us return to a consideration of the civilized people who, being very learned, anxious, and defeatist, mobilize all the scientific and technical means at their disposal in order to destroy symptoms. They come to a tragic end, including that of their own existence.

Palliative medicine is unconcerned with causes and examines only superficial aspects. It refuses to involve the patient, the cause of the disease. As a consequence, I am able to declare here once and for all *that symptomatic medicine will never cure cancer.* Nor will it ever truly cure any disease, not even a common cold.

Non-civilized people, humble and modest, given to self-criticism and confidence in the Order of the Infinite Universe, look to themselves for the cause of their misfortunes. There they find the error, correct it, and re-establish health and peace. Their method of accomplishing this is extremely simple—prayer and fasting. To pray is to view everything in terms of Yin and Yang, the Absolute Justice of the Infinite Universe. To fast is to abjure excess, especially of proteins, relieving the kidneys and liver, and thus generally easing the whole organism. How simple is this essence of the fundamental, divine, and omnipotent medicine!

People of the Western world, why are you blind to the causes of human disease and unhappiness? Why do you rely on destructive means of eliminating only superficial and passing symptoms? Do you not realize that these symptoms, only temporarily repressed, are bound to reappear again in infinitely varied forms?

Consider diabetes: Symptomatic medicine diagnoses it as an insufficiency of insulin. Doctors, therefore, recommend insulin injections. Is this not simplistic and infantile? Doctors do not concern themselves with the *cause* of this insufficiency. Hypo-insulinism (diabetes) (high blood sugar) is always preceded by hyper-insulinism (hypoglycemia) (low blood sugar). If we abundantly and regularly introduce insulin from an external source, the pancreas will grow lazier and lazier and will eventually completely lose its capacity to produce insulin, like a spoiled child used to getting everything he asks for.

Let us consider a second example: Warts and foot corns, both excrescences, are masses of excess protein. *Non-existent in vegetarians,* they affect *females more than males, which means that females have a greater capacity for protein-production than males and must, therefore, remain stricter in their abstention from animal food.* Total suppression of animal protein from the diet causes warts and corns to disappear in a few days without palliative or symptomatic treatment. The same is true of any other tumescent formation caused by excess protein. I have personally observed a case in which a young girl rid herself of approximately two hundred warts on her legs and feet by following the recommendations of our philosophy-medicine for only three weeks, without the help of any external treatment. (Cancer, also, is a proteinic growth.)

And here is a third example—falling hair: In London, on subway-walls and elsewhere, I have often seen advertisements for specialists who claim to know how to remedy falling hair. Yet baldness is exceedingly common in England. Why? What is its cause?

Scientific civilization, unconcerned by the obvious contrast between Europeans and Asians, has never looked for the mechanism that produces hair on the body. But how is it that Europeans, being more hairy, are also more afflicted with baldness? Why is it that, in this connection, no one has ever made significant note of the fact that *Orientals eat very little animal protein?*

Wild herbivorous animals must search constantly for plant-sources of energy. Local and seasonal variations as well as other biological and bioecological circumstances sometimes drastically limit food supply. But being blessed with adaptive functions, which develop in inverse proportion to the poverty of their supply, they are able to build proteins necessary to their species. This great productive capacity, variable and elastic, fluctuates according to nitrogen supply and overall living conditions. In particular, more protein is produced in winter when plant food frequently diminishes, whereas in summer, generally a time of abundance, production is curtailed.

Yin produces Yang, and Yang produces Yin. This is a fundamental law of life that is completely ignored by modern biology and physiology.

You can now understand why wild animals grow fatter in a cold climate, which is apparently hostile and unfavorable. The dialectical adaptability of all wild or natural animals permits production of more protein during winter. Another way of putting it is to say that cold (which is yin) stimulates adaptability and productivity (yang).

Man's discovery of fire and salt marked the beginning of civilization. Fire and salt, two important factors of yangization, enabled man to obtain at will warmth and energy from the outside. As a result, he lost a measure of resistance to cold, eventually being forced to wear clothes. Naturally, the more clothes he wore, the more susceptible to cold he became. This is dialectical logic in dynamic action: *the greater the utility, the greater the inutility.*

Fire and salt, while decreasing man's yang adaptive abilities, also increased the yin side of his nature, resulting in greater sensitivity, sentimentality, and exclusiveness. Growing gradually less capable of producing his own proteins, man turned to more frequent meat-eating in an effort to obtain them. But the more animal proteins he consumes, the more dependent he becomes on lower species. Growing lazier and lazier (in other words, more and more "civilized"), he no longer hunts or even raises cattle for himself. That chore he leaves to the professional cattle-breeder.

So one thing leading to another, man loses almost completely his ability to produce proteins specific to his own nature. He leans more heavily on animal products, which are "tastier" and easier to digest. Consuming greater and greater amounts, his organism is soon driven to mechanisms whereby excess protein can be destroyed and eliminated, thus decreasing the obstructing, if not menacing, heat- and energy-producing reserves. But the breakdown of proteins is accompanied by a significant increase in extra-cellular acidity, which produces general dilation of the organs, tissues, and skin. The rapid discharge of energy manifests itself in immediate and sudden activities: quarrelsome relations or violent and/or excessively frequent sexual relations, which yinnize man through loss of energy and salt. In sum, general yinnization results. Skin, the organ most easily dilated in the body, loses its capacity to hold hair follicles: hence, falling hair.

The immediate and principal cause of baldness is excess sexual activity, which, in turn, springs from a diet too rich in meat. (Another cause of baldness is an excess of vitamin C, sugar, potassium, phosphorus, etc. [all yin factors], which dilate or yinnize tissues and skin.)

Once the cause of falling hair is thus established, the cure is extremely simple: total suppression of sugar and reduced intake of fruits, animal protein, and other yin factors. (Ed. note: although most animal products are yangizing in the short run, they are yinnizing in the long run, because the sodium (yang) in them soon leaves the body, after which the remains of the animal protein turn to very yin acids.) (One-third ounce of seaweed taken daily is also useful. The Japanese favor more than one hundred varieties—of which wakame, hiziki, and arame are the most effective.)

Japanese women who enjoy seaweed use seaweed shampoo made from hunori, and those who avoid meat have beautiful hair reaching quite frequently to a length of five feet. You can still see thick ropes made from their hair several hundred years ago. The ropes were used for hauling blocks of stone from the northern provinces across fields and mountains to Kyoto, the Buddhist capital, where they were used to build the huge Honganji Cathedral, located near the city's central station. In the cathedral today, you can see perhaps ten coils of ropes, each rope four inches in diameter and several yards long, rolled up like extraordinary boas.

And there you have in rough form the basic difference between symptomatic and fundamental medicine. But do not misunderstand—I am not completely denying the usefulness of symptomatic techniques. Our philosophy recognizes and delineates seven stages of judgment and understanding, and the vast majority of people are caught at lower levels, in fact, at the lowest, which we call mechanical or blind. For these, symptomatic and palliative treatment is useful. But for those who wish to live long, complete, magnificent, and amusing lives, and who wish to fulfill their fondest dreams with ease, for these the seventh stage or Supreme Judgment (cosmic consciousness) alone can suffice. The philosophy-medicine of the Far East will serve you as a faithful and reliable guide.

A Criticism of Symptomatic Therapeutics

There are many things I cannot understand in the therapeutics of symptomatic medicine. For instance:

1. *"Cancer is neither a poison nor a parasite which invades us: it is composed of mysterious, malignant cells produced by our own bodies."**

At least Western medicine has discovered that cancer is autogenous. Yet science, so renowned for its precision and exactitude, cannot determine the mechanism of production. I find this failure difficult to explain.

Dr. H., a Japanese medical specialist, states that "the cause of cancer is salt in food, or possibly rice." This specialist is guilty of a double, dualistic mistake:

a. In accusing salt, he attacks the seasoning used most commonly since antiquity in all kitchens of the world prior to the recent importation of sugar. Thus, this doctor must prove that there were many more cancer patients in olden times than there are today (clearly not the case). In addition, he does not understand how salt, acting as a factor of yangization in cooking, can cure cancer.

b. For thousands of years, Japanese as well as Chinese have been

---

* This italicized text, and all those following in the chapter, are taken from *Cancer*, by Dr. W. Nakahara, President of the Cancer Institute of Japan and published by Iwanami (1963, 11th edition).

rice-eaters. Yet cancer was by no means common in these countries in former ages. On the contrary, the rise in the incidence of cancer dates back only a few decades. Moreover, there are two separate and distinct categories of rice: (1) whole ("brown") rice, which is not refined, and can therefore be preserved indefinitely without any chemical treatment; and (2) rice stripped of its transparent, protective hull (which is extraordinarily resistant to all chemical products, including sulfuric acid) and of its several intermediate layers that contain many of the minerals (including calcium), vitamins (especially B vitamins), fats, and proteins that are necessary to man. The polishing of rice reduces it to a muddy starch, a defective, *partial* food that cannot be preserved without the aid of chemicals or special storage. This over-refined rice, called "white rice," has become quite popular since the "Engleburg" machine was imported from Germany some sixty years ago. (In Japan, white rice is known as "Kasu"—waste of rice.)

A man of sensory judgment is a slave to his tastes. His condition is fraught with danger. The decline of world empires, as well as that of any organism, begins from within. Only fearful, exclusive, defeatist, and irresponsible people claim that unhappiness comes from the outside, thus revealing their dependence on external conditions, their state of voluntary slavery. He who accuses another stands accused himself (of his dependence on the other).

The Order of the Infinite Universe, which sustains, animates, destroys, and transmutes everything, the visible and the invisible, is Absolute Justice. All who are not aware of this Absolute Justice must pay a high price.

Dr. H., who accuses salt and rice (both polished and whole) of being causes of cancer, will stand accused himself. He will pay a high price for his error, ending sooner or later like all the great Japanese cancer-specialists: one by one they have perished of cancer, their debt doubly discharged through premature death and loss of face! If you feed whole rice and white rice to a rat, it will always choose the whole rice. It is *never* mistaken. Cancer specialists such as Dr. H. possess much lower judgment than does a rat.

Dr. H. also finds it appropriate to frighten people into drinking milk by claiming that it is essential to human health. His position contradicts the long-held Japanese belief that cow's milk is not a suitable aliment for adults, being destined solely for calves and then only in the few months after birth. The Japanese have always tried to avoid the exploitation of other animals in order to maintain their own human independence. Besides, Dr. H. would be hard-put to show that cancer prevails among those who abstain from the use of milk.

The Japanese accept everything gracefully—bad weather as well as good—and, because of their familial and academic upbringing, have no use for the word "protest." As a consequence, out of loyalty to the Western authorities whom they welcomed unconditionally more than a century ago, they have overcome their repulsion for cow's milk. How difficult this was in the beginning! Giving the milk of a cow to dear babies and children meant making them milk-brothers and sisters of calves, adopted children of animals! This, of course, is but a sentimental objection, but on what *scientific* grounds are Western specialists so much in favor of cow's milk?

Have modern women lost, or do they want to lose, their capacity for lactation? Is breast-feeding so unpopular because of fashion or scientific superstition? Or is modern mercantilism behind the trend? Whatever the reason, man's dependence on animal milk is an alarming development—especially after his full set of teeth have come in.

One can accuse *anything* of being the cause of cancer (milk, salt, rice, even air). But one must explain in detail, biologically and biochemically, the mechanism by which this cancer is produced. At the same time, one must provide a fundamental, effective, and everlasting cure. Otherwise, one's claims are meaningless. Sociological, geographical, and political statistics are of no value in the fields of health, beauty, happiness, justice, and liberty. Moreover, decisions arrived at by statistics, election, or vote of the majority are valid only in a society composed of ignoramuses, slaves, and individuals caught at the lower stages of judgment—in short, people who are unaware of the meaning of justice for man. Majority, as well as authority, can err. History provides many tragic examples: consider such martyrs as Socrates, Jesus, Galileo, Giordano Bruno (burned to death), Martin Luther (accused by the Vatican), as well as the legions of arbitrary scientific masters who have oppressed their brilliant disciples.

Majority equals mass. Mass is physical force. Genius and clairvoyant wisdom can be and often are vested in a minority. Physical force and spiritual force are opposite and sometimes antagonistic. Statistics, the accumulated "wisdom" of the masses, have little to do with intuition and genius. The majority can determine price, but not value.

Let us consider the controversy surrounding cigarettes. The American government, convinced by the statistics of physicians, has declared that smoking is probably the most serious cause of lung cancer. The state has complied with majority opinion—again. (A similar position was maintained between 1919 and 1933 in the government's prohibition of alcohol.) In so-called "democratic" countries, all policies are dominated by the strength of the majority. This condemnation of smoking will end like the "prohibition" that preceded it.

After alcohol was invented in ancient China, the first of its three wise emperors foresaw that much trouble would come of it in the future. But he refused to exercise his powers of prohibition. As a result, the Chinese do not drink much, and there has been very little alcoholism in the country. The judgment of the populace has remained high, thanks to the teaching of the practical and universal dialectics of Yin and Yang.

The warnings blared at American smokers are based only on statistics, not logic. The public remains unenlightened as to the mechanism by which smoking produces lung cancer. Reports have it that some carcinogenic materials are contained in cigarette smoke—but there are more abundant carcinogenic materials of a related nature in the "smog" of London. In fact, in that city everyone breathes a quantity of such contaminants corresponding to the smoking of eighty cigarettes a day.

All arguments on subjects of which next to nothing is known are simply a waste of time. What *would* be relevant would be to give an accurate and precise biological, bio-chemical, and physiological explanation of the mechanism by which cancer occurs in the organisms of smokers and non-smokers alike.*

First, individual differences with regard to natural immunity to cancer must be explained. Even more importantly, we must be clearly told what natural immunity is. Neither modern medicine nor physiology provides an answer but, instead, camouflages ignorance with meaningless terminology. Immunity is "something unknown and incomprehensible"—a worthy counterpart of the "feverish humors" of Molière's medical comedies.

Immunity (resistance to any potential sickness) is a characteristic of health, according to the practical, dialectical philosophy of the Far East. And what is health? It is the normal condition of all living beings. And what is life? It is the materialization of the Infinite-Absolute-Invisible through extended stages of cosmogonic, energetic, nuclear, and atomic organization, followed by geological eras of monocellular and multicellular organization that culminates in man. Inversely, it is the lengthy return trip through dematerialization towards eternal spiritualization. And, thus, "death" is a mere invention of fear, a shadow attached to ignorance of the imposing Order of the Infinite Universe.

According to the Unifying Principle, tobacco smoking is classified as yang. Tobacco grows in warm, yang climates, thereby producing predominantly yin characteristics. The plant is tall, controlled by centrifugal force, and possesses large leaves. While it is growing, then, tobacco is extremely yin. Later, however, it is *dried, dehydrated* (loss of water, which is yin, means yangization) and then it is *burned*. This final means of yangization expels everything yin. The

* (Note: Since this writing, evidence linking smoking with lung cancer has increased; whether this correlation exists if one is using a proper diet and non-chemicalized tobacco remains to be seen. —*Ed.*)

smoke rising upwards from the end of a lighted cigarette is bluish or violet (yin), while that proceeding downwards from the opposite end is a reddish-yellow (yang) color. (Everything that moves toward the center of the earth, for example, is controlled by yang centripetal force.) Scientifically speaking, violet smoke contains yin components, whereas reddish-yellow smoke contains yang components, observations that are perfectly confirmed through biochemical analysis.

Cancer being produced by an excess of protein, it is therefore logical that the yang smoke of tobacco is very much to be recommended in its cure and prevention. Simple observation shows that one loses weight when beginning to smoke (through yangization, constriction, centripetality) while expansive weight-gain accompanies the cessation of smoking. Also, pregnant women who smoke give birth to thinner, smaller babies.

So smoking is yangizing. Cancer—explosive yinnization—is opposed in its development by constricting yang smoke, the effect of which can be a definite regression or even final disappearance of the disease.

Of course, tobacco smoking is not the only means of curing cancer. Many other and more efficient methods exist. But it can very certainly be stated that tobacco smoking in moderate amounts is beneficial for cancer patients as well as for all who wish to strengthen their natural immunity to cancer. (See note page 68.)

2. *"Cancerous cells, like amoebae, are extremely mobile. Because of this, it is extremely difficult to catch and destroy them."*

This feeble excuse is reminiscent of the story of the soldier who complained that his enemy kept moving and refused to present a good target. Movement, instability, and centrifugality are yin characteristics. Nothing is easier to check than such migratory tendencies: simply reduce the daily intake of yin elements, especially sugar but also nuts, fruits, salad, oil, water, animal proteins, and other yinnizing foods.

3. *"Cancerous cells disperse very easily throughout the organism, creating many difficulties."*

Separation and dispersion of cells are yin—confirming once again the extremely yin nature of the disease. When will modern researchers begin to focus their efforts in the proper direction?

4. *"When the end nears, the cancer patient loses protein more and more rapidly; at the same time a mysterious loss of blood occurs."*

All functions develop through being exercised, and protein-storage, which eventuates in cancer, is no exception. It stands to reason that the more one partakes of needless proteins, the more efficient this storage-mechanism will become.

Protein is provided to the body's internal environment by the blood, and blood is manufactured in the intestines from digested food particles. I arrived at this conviction of forty years' standing through application of the incomparable Unifying Principle. In recent years, Professors Chishima and Morishita of Japan succeeded in filming microscopically the transformation of digested food particles into blood and that of red cells into proteinic cancer elements, scientifically substantiating my position and clearly disproving the hypothesis that blood is manufactured in bone marrow—an hypothesis arrived at by observing the change of bone marrow in blood in *sick people.*

The mechanisms that transform digested food particles into blood, and blood into cancer cells, are yin. Both of these transformations can be reversed at will by one who knows how to apply yang factors.

5. *"Cancer is the most dreadful enemy in the history of mankind."*

This exclusive and arrogant statement completely negates the Christian principle, "Do not resist, not even evil." But cancer is not your neighbor or even a tenant in your house. *Cancer is indeed your blood brother!* To react with hostility is to admit fear. Hostility and fear are characteristic of a man who lacks confidence, universal love, and generosity, who is already beaten and defeated. The therapeutics of symptomatic medicine is the corollary of this defeatist mentality.

In order to cure a cancer-patient who has already surrendered, it is first necessary to change his attitude. This must be accomplished at any cost. Otherwise, everything is useless, and the patient might just as well be dead. The case of Dr. Y. Tazaki, head of the hospital attached to the Central Institute of Cancer of Japan, illustrates this point quite well.

Born July 5, 1898, died May 24, 1963, Dr. Tazaki was one of the Directors of the National Movement for Rapid Detection of Cancer. His own cancer of the gum was discovered two years prior to his death while it was still only the size of a grain of rice. He immediately wrote his will, which was published soon after his death in a popular monthly magazine, "Hujin Koron." Reading it shocked me deeply, and I deplore it as a representation of Western authoritative medicine:

Will—August 28, 1961

My case must not be publicized as a case of cancer, but rather as a chronic inflammation of the gum. I request this on behalf of my two daughters who are still quite young. (I fear that my condition may decrease their chances of getting married.)

Still another reason not to mention the word "cancer" is that for years I have worked to propagate throughout Japan the idea that "the quicker the detection, the more certain the cure." So people must not learn that I was unable to cure myself. So many would become discouraged and would lose confidence in the efficacy of modern medicine.

In my opinion, cancer cannot be controlled, and it often appears in parts of the body where no chronic irritation has occurred.

The patient must never be told he has cancer. If he is himself a doctor, great caution should be exercised as to the terminology used when speaking to him.

Judging by his will, it is clear that Dr. Tazaki was not a true scientist, that he was a fatalist, and that he thought it impossible to cure cancer—in short, that he possessed a self-defeating mentality. He was tragically afraid.

6. *"Researchers have learned how to produce cancer artificially."*

In 1915, and for the first time in history, Dr. Yamagiwa succeeded in artificially inducing cancer in a mouse after sacrificing about 12,000 of the animals. He rubbed tar on their skin in order to prove his hypothesis that cancer arises where there is chronic irritation. Later, he founded the Cancer Institute of Japan.

I admire Dr. Yamagiwa's patience and his will to succeed, but I cannot appreciate his experimental method, which was more empirical than logical.

From the very beginning, research on cancer has been based on statistics. If a certain number of workmen developed cancer, it was immediately concluded that the materials they handled daily must have contained carcinogenic chemical components. What simplistic thinking! How absurd! When it is proved that contact with a certain product can result in cancer, one has not yet determined whether it was the chemical composition of the product or irritation that was actually responsible. Even after this point has been satisfactorily clarified, one must still consider all the physical, biological, chemical, and physiological ramifications, as well as *other variables* such as the professional field, sex and age of the individual, the season, locale, and climate, etc. When all these preconditions to a thorough scientific investigation have been met, one must still determine if there might not be exceptions—individuals possessing natural immunity. Should only one of these be found, a researcher would have to begin again at the beginning, unravelling the threads of this new mystery.

Alas for medicine! Doctors are satisfied after having fulfilled empirically and conceptually *only a single one* of these prerequisites. They ignore the part played by each of the others, even that of natural immunity, the existence of which is well-established nowadays.

In recent times, many varieties of cancer have been produced artificially—by Bashford, Flexner-Jobling, Hujinami Likubo, Kato, Yoshida, etc. It is not known if these cancers are related, why they are produced by different chemical compounds, through what mechanisms they appear, why some of them can be transplanted and continue their development in healthy animals whereas others cannot, and so forth. A great many problems crave solution.

Examined in the light of the dialectical and practical Unifying Principle, all chemical substances with which one succeeds in producing cancer (such as quinine, fructose, rhodamine, nitrogenous coloring agents, etc.) reveal themselves to be *extremely yin.*

7. *"While studying cancer in mice, E. Bashford and M. Haarand found that it was possible to immunize these animals with injections of cells from healthy animals of the same specie, and that, in particular, the skin of a fetus and whole blood were especially efficacious."*

Healthy cells, young bloods cells (particularly those of a fetus), and whole blood are all yang. What else do Bashford and Haarand need to know?

8. *"Although it has heretofore been thought impossible, cancer can be transplanted from one animal to another of a different species if the latter has first been sufficiently radiated with x-rays."*

Yes, x-rays are *extremely* yinnizing!

9. *"Dr. Sirai demonstrated that a heterogenous cancer can be transplanted into the brain."*

This is evident if one takes into consideration the fact that the brain is the organ that maintains itself in the most yin condition—as opposed to the sole of the foot that, on the contrary, maintains the most yang condition. By the same token, we should point out to Dr. Sirai that the sole of the foot is the part of the body most resistant to heterogenous implantation of cancer, especially if the foot is not "flat." As might be expected, the organs most open to heterogenous implantation are yin—the eye and the skin in general.

10. *"The theory that cancer is caused by a virus is more and more frequently held nowadays."*

Despite the popular saying to the contrary, fiction is stranger than truth—at least when investigators of reality possess dim imaginations and fix upon any plausible suspect as an excuse to abandon the chase. The virus—invisible, unknown, and possibly non-existent—possesses the qualification of the perfect suspect: it cannot defend itself. It has been framed by doctors who are incapable of tracking down the real culprit. As for the comical theory of a "latent virus," it is like believing in an elusive ghost one thinks one sees but can never quite capture on film.

11. *"One can easily induce cancer of the liver by adding a nitrogenous coloring agent to a rat's food. However, this result cannot be obtained with guinea pigs or rabbits."*

Why? Is it such a mystery? Must one resort to the theory of a "latent" or "undiscoverable" virus in order to solve the puzzle?

Ignorance willingly perpetuated through lazy imprecision is the same as arrogance or exclusiveness. It requires considerable talent to overlook so obvious a difference as exists between rats and rabbits. The former, being night animals, are yang, while rabbits and guinea pigs, day animals, are exclusively vegetarian, soft-tempered in the extreme, and thus very yin. They would repel, whereas rats would not, a yin chemical product such as a nitrogenous coloring agent.

A similar misunderstanding has confused physiologists with respect to the antagonism that exists between the orthosympathetic (yin) and para-sympathetic (yang) divisions of the autonomic nervous system, especially as these affect the various yin or yang organs. Cancer specialists do not seem to understand even the rudiments of biology and zoology.

12. *"Cancers, artificially produced by the methods of Nishiyama (glucose), W. C. Heuper (nickel), Sakurada (coloring agents) and B. S. and E. T. Oppenheimer (multi-molecular chemical products) can appear in the shape of sarcomas. Although different, these chemicals*

produce identical results. While this might seem totally incomprehensible, the situation can be clarified by postulating the existence of a "latent virus."

One could not more convincingly admit that the concept of a "latent virus" is but a hypothesis of the lowest credibility.

13. *"One can imagine that a cancer virus would exhibit the following characteristics:*
   a. *it would invariably be found in animals subject to the development of cancer;*
   b. *each type of cancer would develop from a particular virus, and each virus would possess distinct characteristics;*
   c. *the various viruses would produce identical cancers according to the species of the animal;*
   d. *the "latent virus" would be activated by a certain metamorphosis of cells (but this would not necessarily be common)."*

Because the "latent virus" does not exist, the search for it will hopefully stop short of despair and desperation. Yet what a tragic and sad perspective it is—so many researchers bogged down in hopeless speculation.

14. *"Most difficult to understand is the fact that sarcomas can result from multi-molecular chemical products hidden in the organism for more than a year. This observation is totally perplexing."*

It would not be perplexing if it were understood that there are yin and yang multi-molecules. With the most yang and the most yin, completely opposed results would naturally be obtained.

15. *"R. Sasaki and T. Yoshida succeeded in producing cancer in rats by administering ortho-amino-azotulene for 250 to 300 days. Without exception, all rats developed cancer under these conditions... R. Kinoshita found that this cancer can be produced with the cream of butter in 150 days."*

In other words, these results parallel those derived from the feeding of nitrogenous coloring agents.

16. *"Cancer can be produced by "kangri" (yang) as well as x-rays, radium, and ultra-violet radiations (yin)."*

It should be remembered that *the same result can be obtained with two antagonistic factors.* For example, the skin can be burned by contact with a very cold object as well as with fire.

17. *"Cancer can be controlled or prevented through administration of liver powder."*

According to dialectical medicine, the liver is one of the five most yang organs, and cancer is an excess of yin. Even Pearl Buck's mother knew of this remedy (see her novel, *The Mother*).

18. *"Professor Nagayo was unanimously elected first president of the Cancer Institute of Japan. Two months later, in June, he became ill; it was diagnosed as cancer; he died on August 16 of the same year. Professor Nishina, a famed scientist of cancer, also developed liver cancer and died within two months. Liver cancer is the most serious type and, for the time being, it does not respond to any known treatment."*

(Dr. Y. Tazaki, director of the National Cancer Hospital, and Dr. T. Tamiya, president of the National Cancer Center, have also died of cancer.)

Nearly everyone has known for a long time that liver powder is especially efficacious in the prevention and control of cancer. Yet not a single specialist has endeavored to discover why. Is this laziness, carelessness, incapacity, or scientific blindness? Can doctors, who monopolize a profession vital to the whole of humanity, continue to remain utterly ignorant? Are they not aware of their responsibility, their duty to think and to practice self-criticism? Had the first emperors of China heard of such irresponsibility, they would have had all doctors burned or buried alive. And if the President of the United States had had good sense, instead of endorsing the national campaign against cigarettes, he would immediately abolish the entire medical establishment.

19. *"According to Dr. F. R. White, the nitrogen content of cancerous cells does not diminish when the animal receives an alimentation nearly or completely devoid of nitrogen. This means that cancerous cells take nitrogen from the animal for their development."*

Having read one of Terroine's three volumes (published in 1933), and especially the chapter entitled, "Is Nitrogen Disappearing?," one is compelled to think through the entire question of protein-development. Terroine examined fifty-one discourses published by various authors.

Another writer, Louis Kervran, who published *Biological Transmutations* in 1962, set forth scientifically proven principles of change that operate within the living organism, which explain the nitrogen-transfer mechanism Dr. Nakahara seeks to understand in the above quotation.

20. *"The behavior of cancerous cells is not dependent upon oxygen-supply."*

This is yet another confirmation of the fact that cancer is a storage of excess yin factors. Because cancer is yin, it does not need oxygen (also yin).

21. *"In the United States, 220,000 persons die of cancer each year. Seventy thousand consulting cancer patients are saved. The rate of attrition would be greatly reduced if anti-cancerous institutions were in a higher state of development."*

This is at best a pious hope in an unlikely hypothesis. We can only wish Dr. Nakahara good luck. Once the real cause of cancer has been recognized, hostility toward the disease will disappear.

We have had ample opportunity in this chapter to examine the exclusive mentality of modern medicine, which destroys microbes and viruses in an effort to establish a germ-free world, a world without evil or evildoer. Can it not observe that good and evil, wrongdoer and benefactor, are two equally necessary aspects of Life (Oneness).

The Virus

Nuclear science has found that matter is non-matter, and that

Energy comes from nowhere.

"Nonsense!" despaired Professor Bridgman—

Before taking his life...

Scientific medicine finally discovered the ultimate killer

Of all mankind.

Visible and invisible, physical and metaphysical.

At the same time life and death, existing and non-existent.

The Virus!

Ghost and nightmare of symptomatic medicine,

It engrosses thousands of helpless doctors who search in

Fascination, amazement... despair.

Will it swallow up the whole of medicine?

Eventually, man will turn his eyes from the microscope

To the macrocosm, and

Contemplate

The limitless horizons

Of the Infinite Universe.

Man will owe to the virus a new medicine—

Fundamental and divine,

Omnipotent and omniscient.

It will deal with life and man,

Not analytically, not dualistically,

But with Universal

Understanding.

Dialectical Medicine

Above mountains of white, brilliant clouds (dark with uncertainty and fear for those looking up from below), I amuse myself in contemplation of a superb view of the Infinite, free of the frames of reference of time and space. I am sitting comfortably on a small Oriental flying carpet. I can see East and West, past and future, reflected on the screen of a little pocket transistor-television manufactured millions and millions of years ago and called "imagination."

The scenes unfolding on earth are intriguing. In the West, I am witnessing the finale of *"Scientific and Technical Civilization."* A very animated, chaotic ending it is, extremely complicated and distressing to the participants, leading at the conclusion to nuclear debate. In the East, it is intermission time; the curtain has been lowered, the actors who are to play *"The Awakening Dragon"* are sleeping soundly, exhausted after having performed so long *"Light from the Orient"* and *"Colonization."*

Next will come *"Universal Peace."* Everyone is waiting. When will the curtain lift? Let us look at our little transistor-television to see what has gone before:

Five thousand years ago, two independent civilizations reigned on earth. One in the East, the other in the West, they were monistic, religious, and industrious. The Western civilization was subdued approximately two thousand years ago by a forceful, dualistic society born on the shores of the Mediterranean.

But all visible and invisible phenomena have a beginning and *end.*

For reasons of balance (opposites attracting one another), the newborn civilization of force required a proper moral teaching and imported an Eastern philosophy of peace and love (Christianity), which facilitated the rule and eventual enslavement of its ignorant, obedient, and generally industrious populace.

Eventually the civilization of physical force, having gained control through conquest of the entire ancient world, established an *"Empire of Abundance and Abuse."* Abundance and abuse, however, produced laziness, weakening the conquerors, diluting their strength.

So, in turn, the civilization of physical force disappeared, leaving behind its moral precepts in a form called *"Christianity,"* which dominated the western world for some time, benefitting from the material and political remnants of the fallen empire. But, naturally, its own hour of darkness also came. And the world was left in gloom.

In time, a new dualistic school appeared, grew rapidly amidst challenges and sacrifices, and succeeded in sweeping away all that remained of the former religious hegemony. This new dualism was called *"Science and Technology."* Having eliminated the spiritual, it sought to dominate the physical. It explored matter thoroughly, down through the nuclear level, striving to consolidate its victory on a permanent basis. But in this relative and finite world, "all visible and invisible phenomena have a front and a back." *"Science and Technology"* began to suffer at the hands of its own offspring— *"Money."*

Now, *"Money"* thrives, controlling industry and commerce. It inspires organizations that are, in effect, reincarnated feudal kings. These organizations join in defensive and offensive alliances designed to monopolize Prince *"Money."* New struggles begin. The conqueror becomes the conquered, as always...

Today, another wrestler is entering the ring: *"The Worker."* ("The last becomes first.") Soon, however, having achieved dominion, the worker will succumb in turn, assassinated by his nemesis: *"Disease."* Consider its *"Army"*: cancer, allergy, heart disease, diabetes; and its *"Navy"*: epilepsy, schizophrenia, paranoia. Who can protect himself?

Most to be dreaded is madness, because it leads to the manufacture of ever more powerful weapons of destruction. At the same time, it clouds the Supreme Judgment. Its most effective tool is food, which can kill accurately and precisely, snaring the individual on his own hook—blind and sensorial greed.

The civilization of the Far East, however, playing *"Light from the Orient,"* has long shown the way. Its own people have lived in peace, quietly and piously—obedient, submissive, honest, and industrious. But the law of beginning and end rules everywhere—dispassionately and impartially. Throughout the centuries, Orientals grew softer and softer, always graceful, never protesting, accepting everything with thankfulness and joy, so that eventually their countries were overrun and colonized. Joining the Western camp, they fight dualistically alongside their conquerors against *"Disease."*

Nowadays, the scientific, technological civilization rules supreme. But its medicine, controlled by money, can attack only symptoms and exterior manifestations, avoiding the cause of the disease itself. If symptomatic medicine does not undergo reform, it will be the ruination of mankind.

Civilizations as well as individuals—macrocosms and microcosms—lose happiness and life when they become arrogant, exclusive and domineering. Dualists ignore the law of beginning and end. That is why all dictatorial civilizations have vanished one after another.

Only the beginningless does not end: the Order of the Infinite Universe (God in Western antiquity), Absolute Justice, Infinite Freedom, Universal Supreme Judgment, Love, the All-Embracing, Divine Grace, and so on. All these names refer to one thing only: Life. Life is the Order of the Infinite Universe, which perpetually animates and transmutes everything in this finite and relative world. Life is omnipotent, omniscient, and omnipresent.

Unfortunately, scientific and technical medicine is not based on awareness of Life. Consequently, it cannot cure disease. Instead it employs destructive weaponry: radium, war, gas, x-rays, radioactive cobalt, neutrons. Whatever destroys well is well-received. Modern

Western medicine does not see that the symptoms of disease are the most useful alarms Life has bequeathed us.

Eastern medicine, respectful toward Universal Life and therefore completely alien to the Western viewpoint, is dialectical, logical, and fundamental. It does not attack symptoms, which are merely superficial. (Of course, it does not deny the efficacy of certain symptomatic treatments, but it relegates these to a role of secondary importance.) Its basic approach is nutritional and educative. First and foremost, it is a philosophical school in which one learns the secret of longevity and happiness, free of dependence upon doctors.

As a branch of philosophy, Eastern medicine does not accept the idea of an "incurable" disease. Mainly in Japan I have studied, practiced, and taught its principles for fifty years. On my sixtieth birthday, leaving my homeland in order to determine whether there might be some country on earth where this philosophy-medicine would be neither applicable nor efficient, I went to India. There I encountered many diseases unknown in Japan: leprosy, leucoderma, Hodgkin's disease, etc.—all supposedly "incurable" by scientific methods, but curable by ours.

I also journeyed to Black Africa, to Lambaréné, to meet Dr. Albert Schweitzer and help him, if possible, for the rest of my life. At that time, I did not know that he was only a surgeon who had studied the most symptomatic of medicines in order to be welcomed in Black Africa as a "witch doctor." He hadn't the faintest notion of a dialectical and monistic philosophy of Life. He killed billions of microbes daily and dumped the refuse from his surgical procedures in the holy Ogooue River. His operations and amputations caused me many sleepless nights as I lay awake, listening to the screaming of his victims.

I began to teach the method of curing diseases without amputating limbs, without employing drugs, but rather through the use and appreciation of natural foods in natural proportions. Epilepsy, Hodgkin's disease, leprosy, tropical ulcers, asthma—all terrible equatorial diseases—were cured without difficulty. Patients came to me more frequently. Moving to the Protestant Mission of Dindende, one and a half miles upstream on the holy river, I was given an old cottage which, forty years ago, had served as Dr. Schweitzer's residence and hospital. The black people followed. Newcomers arrived from far and near, traveling in little canoes as much as 125 miles. Every morning, opening the windows, I was confronted with a crowd of black men and women, young and old alike. One morning, I heard that nobody was calling that day at the Great Doctor's clinic: all patients had come to Dindende.

It could not go on like this. My wife and I were only two, while approximately forty worked at the hospital. Deciding to stop my consultations, I dismissed all the patients.

Next morning, opening the window, I found the yard deserted. Jotsuna and I took a walk for the first time in weeks, but were suddenly surrounded on all sides by Negroes who appeared as if by magic from the jungle. Another battalion of them had hidden underneath the house, spending the night there quietly. What could I do?

A chief came to call. At the outset, he asked me to remain. "We will build you a hospital to your specifications, just as we did for the Great Doctor."

I said that it might be impossible for me to stay.

"But we used to have much better health," he went on, "about thirty-five years ago. It was only after the Great Doctor came that we grew so weak. Many of the diseases we have now were completely unknown in the old days. Already, three tribes have completely disappeared. The Great Doctor has brought wine, condensed milk, and medications—many bad things. Half of our friends who go to the hospital come out amputated—crippled for life. The other half seem to remain there, either hospitalized or working as servants or nursing aids, cooks, or carpenters. We've become slaves because of medicine. But you don't use medicine, and you don't amputate. You teach us how and what to eat in order to cure ourselves. You must remain with us always."

His childlike and sincere simplicity moved us so deeply that even Jotsuna would have liked me to remain forever. But as was explained in the Introduction to this book, a sad event obliged us to leave these adorable friends.

In Black Africa, I saw multitudinous errors attributable to the techniques of symptomatic medicine: iatrogenic diseases, mistaken diagnoses, unnecessary amputations... Just one example among many was the attitude of white doctors who claimed that sexual activity among blacks was undeterred by morality, almost the entire population supposedly suffering from gonorrhea, for which painful treatments were prescribed. One could hear the desperate screams of the patients every day in the small village of Lambaréné.

But in reality these were *not* cases of gonorrhea. Moreover, among the small native population, there were no prostitutes. Eating a great deal of fruit rich in vitamin C (mangoes, avocados, etc.) produced an inflammation of the urethra, and often of the bladder itself, the symptoms closely resembling those of gonorrhea.

I have seen hell in action in the jungles of Africa. The differences between white and black mentalities, their fundamental misunderstandings, stand out clearly there. Essentially, the distinction is as between East and West. A unifying view of the world, a philosophy that has been strongly monistic for several thousands of years, is now practically extinct due to colonization. In its turn, the dualistic philosophy prevalent among white people for approximately two thousand years must now be completely reassessed in light of the discoveries of nuclear science. The principles and laws of experimental science, once conceived of as definitive, now stand on tottering foundations! Whites and blacks alike find themselves in a blind alley.

This is why the philosophy-medicine of the Far East should be reconsidered today. Almost totally forgotten by Orientals themselves, it is difficult for civilized peoples to understand without the assistance of a competent guide. (And these are few and far between nowadays.)

This medicine-philosophy leads to awareness of Infinite Freedom, Eternal Happiness, and Absolute Justice. In the sphere of family and social relations, this awareness is experienced as peace. The method is simple—daily practice, which can be in terms of diet, intellectual understanding, or, preferably, both.

First, we must define health. According to our medicine-philosophy, it is characterized by the following properties:

1. ABSENCE OF FATIGUE, such as that of a primitive man who can run all day on the trail of an animal, stopping only because he is hungry, never because he is tired.

2. GOOD APPETITE, expressed in terms of hunger that is satisfied with *either* "gourmet" eating *or* the simplest dishes, all of which are enjoyed with great gratitude.

3. SOUND SLEEP, entered into in three minutes at any time and place; devoid of movement and dreams—especially nightmares; and awakening at a predetermined time with instant, full alertness, like a lion pouncing on a rabbit. If a man sleeps more than six hours, he is lazy, if not diseased. Three to four hours of sleep are more than sufficient for those in good health. Over-sleeping is a waste of time. If you wish to enjoy a long sleep, you will have plenty of opportunity after your death.

The above physiological conditions are worth 5 points each.

4. GOOD MEMORY, "forgetting" nothing. This is very important. Good memory is fundamental to happiness and to our very existence. Without memory, we have no judgment. Without judgment we cannot live a happy and amusing life.

5. LACK OF ANGER, even when you are the target of nasty and sordid accusations, or attacks or criticisms aimed at belittling you.

6. CLARITY AND PROMPTNESS OF THOUGHT AND ACTION, those who are quick, precise, and prepared to answer any challenge are healthy, distinguishing themselves by an ability to establish order everywhere. This orderliness, observable throughout the animal and vegetable kingdoms, is an expression of beauty in action and form. Health and happiness in our daily lives are also expressions of beauty.

The above mental and psychological conditions are worth 10 points each.

7. SENSE OF JUSTICE FOR MAN, if your country's population

is 100,000,000 and the apple-production is limited to 100,000,000 per annum, then you should eat only one apple per year. If for example, in such a case, you eat one apple a day, you encroach upon the rights of 364 of neighbors or compatriots, either through direct violent force or under a masked monetary form. Thus, according to this view of justice, you are a criminal. You are, directly or indirectly, dishonest with your fellow man.

If you understand justice for man and live by it, allow yourself 55 points. When totaling your points, as you approach 100, you are approaching awareness of Eternal Happiness, Infinite Freedom, and Absolute Justice. Notice, however, that from the standpoint of awareness of these absolutes, one is aware of them as absolutes or not at all, whereas in terms of individual health itself, there are degrees.

You can attain health through practice of the dietetic philosophy-medicine that I call "macrobiotics." Since I began teaching it fifty years ago, several *million* copies of my various publications have been sold.

Remember that comprehension and application of our philosophy-medicine not only leads to physical health but also opens wide the gates to awareness of Eternal Happiness, Infinite Freedom, and Absolute Justice. You are even protected against "accidents" because it unveils our extrasensory perception or clairvoyance. (Many testimonials of such unveiling exist in Japan as well as in Europe and America, but it is better for you to experience and learn for yourself so that your understanding will be deepened. Simply practice this philosophy for a couple of weeks, sufficient time to assimilate the basic principles, and verify the value of this practical way of life.)

In Chapter Four *(Miracles)*, I outlined in brief the fifteen basic schools that utilize our dialectical-monistic philosophy in Japan alone. Needless to say, this little book can serve only as a letter of introduction to the magnificent world that gave birth to so many schools.

Our dialectical and practical medicine, however, can be reduced to one simple phrase: justice for man. This concept should not call to mind the image of the courthouse prevalent in so many Western countries: a square, cold, rigid building, severe-looking from the outside and somber, cold, nasty, and cruel within. Justice, as understood in the East, is joyful, familiar, kind, and amusing. Justice for man comes from Absolute Justice: all-embracing Love, Divine Love. Absolute Justice is the impartial law that applies to all that exists. It is the Order of the Infinite Universe, which creates, animates, and transmutes everything. It is the spirit of all existence. It is the quintessence of the Infinite Universe, Life. Absolute Justice provides everything for us. It makes no exceptions and omits nothing. It gives us "bad" weather as well as "good," cold as well as heat, scarcity as well as abundance, difficulty as well as ease, "enemy" as well as friend.

Absolute Justice is absolutely impartial; and he who knows this is also impartial. (However, if you have very strong preferences, it is wiser, in making a choice, to seek a proper balance between yin and yang. In the Orient, it has long been thought that no more virtuous attempt is possible in life.)

The familial, scholastic, social, cultural, scientific, and technical education of the Orient concentrates on teaching methods whereby one can recognize and attain true balance. This education begins at the dinner table, not only from the very first day of a child's existence on this planet but nine months before birth or even earlier still.

Oriental education is fundamental, biological, physiological, and, above all, embryological. You can well imagine that health derived from such an education would be soundly based, that a family built by those who enjoy such health would be happy indeed, that a society composed of such families would be strong, and that world peace can only be established by such societies working in unison.

At any rate, this sociology is fundamental to Oriental principles of government.

But now that the yin, feminine East has been invaded, colonized, and virtually destroyed by the yang, masculine West, the time has come to resurrect its ancient practical wisdom, as found in the great books of the sages: the *I Ching, Vedas, Tao Teh Ching, Charaka*

Samita, Code of Manu, Somon Reisu, Bhagavad Gita, etc.

And what is the mentality of a nation whose way of life is based on such wisdom? It is what Lèvy-Bruhl has called the "primitive mentality." (Forty years ago, I read his books and was so impressed by them that I could not resist traveling to France and calling on this great master of philosophy. But I was shocked to find that his homeland, and the West in general, regarded our traditional "primitive" wisdom as completely incomprehensible.)

The fundamental philosophy of the non-civilized primitive peoples is very simple: accept everything gratefully and without the slightest protest. This is true modesty: *unconditional humiliation;* the "self" recognized as small, ignorant, dishonest, greedy, and miserable. Without such understanding, no human being can attain awareness of the true Self (Oneness). (The "civilized" people I have met, almost without exception, have considered themselves great, wise, honest, generous, and happy.)

To accept everything humbly and unconditionally is to express confidence in Absolute Justice, which does not bring us sickness and anguish to torment us but to reveal to our limited understanding the errors we have made in our ignorance. "If a man is not happy, it is his own fault."

Gratitude and faith are virtual synonyms. Gratitude is deep joy, and faith is deep confidence. He who does not feel and express complete confidence in Absolute Justice is ignorant; and ignorance is the cause of all disease, anxiety, and "accidents." "For what is not of faith is sin." (Romans: 14; 23).

Also in the Bible we read:

Blessed are the meek, for they shall inherit the earth... You have heard it said: 'An eye for an eye and a tooth for a tooth'; but I say to you: 'Resist not, even evil. If someone hits you on the right cheek, turn to him also the left. And if any man takes your coat, give him also your cloak.' ...You have heard it said: 'Love your neighbor and hate your enemy'; but I say to you: 'Love your enemies, bless them that curse you, do good to them that hate you, and pray for them that spitefully

use you or persecute you, for your Father in Heaven makes the sun to
rise on the good *and* on the evil, and he sends rain falling on the just
and on the unjust. Be like your Father in Heaven.'" (Matthew 5: 5, 38-
40, 43-45, 48).

Judge not, that you not be judged... And why do you notice the speck
in your brother's eye, but not the log in your own? Hypocrite! First remove the log from your own eye, and then you will see clearly enough
to remove the speck from your brother's eye. (Matthew: 7; 1, 3-5)

How faithful the "primitive" peoples have been to these teachings! And how quickly they have lost their lands to the conquering
whites... But I advise you this, my dear friends: Imitate these primitives—gracefully give away your home, your land, even your country. You will lose nothing at all. And if new "civilized" men come
from Mars and ask you for the earth, give it with the greatest joy. You
have nothing to lose, because you cannot lose what was never yours
in the first place. Everything you call "mine" will eventually be lost
to you, for there is nothing permanent in this constantly changing
world—nothing, that is, except Change itself, the only constant.

Give everything, and ask for nothing, because everything you
have has been given to you, including your life.

I humbly offer the following prayer for your consideration:

Magnificent is Thy Name.
We are in You.
Everything is realized exactly as You wish it,
On earth and everywhere else,
All the time.
You give us our daily bread.
You give us everything.
Give us more temptations,
And throw us into the hands of the wicked!

This daily prayer is a little different from the Biblical version. But as rewritten by my Western friends in the French study camp last summer, it probably approximates the original, which, over the centuries, was rewritten by Western Gentiles. The Bible (as we know it today) is filled with many contradictions.

Reduced to its essence, the above prayer amounts to a deeply grateful recognition of the Absolute Justice of the Order of the Infinite Universe at all levels of our daily life. Venerating the sublime constitution of Life as the foundation of love and the very fountain of life, we realize that we are wealthier than if we possessed the largest diamond in the world. We realize that to ask for health, freedom, or unveiled judgment is to admit that we know little or nothing about Absolute Justice.

Because we are heirs to the entire Infinite Universe (Life, which includes life and death), we need never kill—not even in "self-defense." There truly is *no enemy anywhere in the Infinite Universe.* Cancer, allergies, heart disease, mental illness, crime, and even capitalistic imperialism are all amusements with which our invisible Producer-Director-Instructor (Oneness) continually confronts us and, thereby, reveals Itself to us.

Why do civilized people consider such trials insufferable or "unjust"? Why are they so exclusive?

Night unfolds. A solitary old man with yellow skin is meditating in a bamboo room. He envisions all his civilized friends whom he loves so dearly, and he thinks... Why do they entangle themselves in violent arguments? Why has the scientific and technical civilization produced so much fear and uncertainty?...

In Tokyo, there lives a certain Dr. Aimi. Now 60 years of age, he has studied symptomatic medicine at Keio University, maintained a practice until the age of 47, and finally abandoned it altogether in favor of the study of Christianity at a Protestant school from which he graduated at the age of 50. Since then, he has cared for patients as a minister and has succeeded in curing many "incurable" diseases by teaching and practicing the medicine of Jesus: the medicine of love. Dr. Aimi has published several books, including *The Key to Miracu-*

lous Cure (a best-seller), is in demand all over Japan as a lecturer, and has thousands of followers.

He explains the mechanisms of miraculous cure in terms of the theories of Selye and Reilly—who are, I believe, the foremost medical scientists in the West today, after Claude Bernard.

Selye's Revolutionary Theory

In 1855, Pasteur found that many bacteria are pathogenic (capable of invading an organism and living on it as parasites). In 1892, Koch discovered the tuberculosis germ; since then, medical scientists and doctors have discovered many germs that can cause disease. But the mechanism by which they produce symptoms, as well as that of immunity to such microbes, remain a mystery to them. Bacteriological pathology has no solid foundation.

According to the theory of Selye, on the other hand, one never becomes diseased if the interbrain (the center of sensitivity and adaptability, composed of the thalamus and hypothalamus) is in good health—resistant to all "stress." Now, if this is true, then he who knows permanent psychic peace, thanks to a religious or moral teaching, will never become diseased, or at the very least will be able to restore very quickly any damage to the body if he does fall ill. (Thus, Dr. Aimi establishes the emotional peace of his patients by using the Bible—and he is very successful in curing not only physical disease but also mental and spiritual anguish. The fact is that Dr. Selye's theory has been understood and practiced in the East for hundreds of years. The word "disease," in both Chinese and Japanese, means "disequilibrium of mind and emotion.")

Dr. Selye is thus correct, in theory. But in practice he insists, as a symptomatic doctor, on the administration of a renal hormone (cortisone) in order to establish the mental peace of the patient. He does not try to discover how to activate the mechanism of the adrenal glands, so that they will produce enough hormones *under any circumstances.*

Thousands of years ago, the dialectical philosophy-medicine revealed the cause of adrenal dysfunction and prescribed the cure:

macrobiotics: natural foods in natural proportions.

Reilly's Theory

I know of only four great scientists of biology and physiology in the West: (1) Claude Bernard; (2) Professor R. Quinton, who devoted his life to research on seawater and eventually came to the conclusion that all living creatures on earth originated in the ocean; (3) L. Kervran, author of the wonderful *Biological Transmutations*, and (4) Professor Reilly. These four (as opposed to such dualists as Aschoff, Pasteur, and Madame Curie) developed monistic theories. Turning their backs on dualistic modern Western science, they looked for something deeper and more fundamental—at least initially. (Unfortunately, being children of Western Aristotelian, Cartesian systems of logic, they eventually returned to dualism.)

In May of 1954, Reilly delivered the results of his lengthy studies to the Societe Biologique de France. His remarkable theories were that:

1. There are no specific germs for any disease.
2. A germ can serve as a mechanical stimulant only to the orthosympathetic nervous system.
3. Symptoms of tuberculosis, diphtheria, typhoid fever, etc. can be produced not only by certain varieties of germs, but also by a pair of tweezers or an electric needle used to excite certain points on the orthosympathetic nerves.

(These statements undermined the very bases of bacteriology and pathology more thoroughly even than did the theory of Selye.) Moreover, Reilly added:

4. Man can be immunized against any "germ-caused" disease by paralyzing or destroying the orthosympathetic nervous system; this can be accomplished surgically or through use of a drug such as chlorpromazine.
5. Most important is the balance and proper functioning of the orthosympathetic nervous system which, when in an ultra-sensitive (yin) state, leaves the organism vulnerable to all germs.

Is not Reilly's theory magnificent? It shows that the origin of disease is not external but internal. We ourselves and not the germs are the cause of our own diseases.

So far, Reilly was correct; unfortunately, his judgment failed to remain so high.

In 1883, Koch created a sensation by declaring that he had discovered the cholera bacillus. In a subsequent demonstration-discussion, Pettenkofer and one of his disciples swallowed a glass of cholera bacilli to disprove Koch's theory. Pettenkofer survived, but his disciple died. Why? Because the great hygienist had, unlike his disciple, a very yang constitution and an extremely strong sympathetic system. The disciple, however, was afraid, which overexcited his sympathetic nerve. Pettenkofer's interbrain, in good condition, was not under "stress."

It is now well understood that if the interbrain and sympathetic system are in good health, we can resist any "attack." Neither invasion of microbes nor stress occurs.

How can one develop a sturdy sympathetic system and interbrain? Only hunger and thirst, difficulties, painful work, cold *and heat* can strengthen these systems. They must be trained from early childhood, as early as the embryological period—such are the teachings of the philosophy of the Far East. All great men were born of industrious, honest mothers who suffered many hardships, especially during pregnancy.

Reilly's research was quite advanced. He discovered that metallic poisons such as sulphur, arsenic, nickel, lead, cobalt, and nicotine can do no harm to the body if the sympathetic system has first been treated with chlorpromazine. But his ideas were known thousands of years ago in the Orient, and even in the country of Christianity, far from the center of civilization:

> And these signs shall follow them that believe; in my name shall they cast out devils; they shall speak with new tongues; they shall take up serpents; and *if they drink any deadly thing, it shall not hurt them;* they shall lay hands on the sick, and they shall recover." (Mark 16: 17-18)

What a pity that Reilly and Selye, being children of Western philosophy, turned their backs at this point, and returned to symptomatic treatments. Reilly recommended immunizing oneself with chlorpromazine to *paralyze* the orthosympathetic nervous system. Instead, he should have advocated means of *strengthening* the nerves, as all wild animals do. Consider the crocodile of Black Africa, who lives so joyfully in a dirty river full of germs and viruses. It can hardly be said to be under "stress." And during the First World War, there were fewer casualties when antibiotics and medications were in short supply than in the modern hospitals of the United States and Canada. The abundance and abuse of antibiotics destroys.

The Constancy of Inconstancy

Everything is inconstant in this relative world, and this inconstancy is the only constancy. That is why life is so amusing, so interesting. The constancy of inconstancy—what a big discovery! By comparison, all other discoveries of man are nothing—including the discovery of America, of Uranus and Pluto, of radium and plutonium, of the hypothetical law of "universal magnetism," and of "$E=mc^2$." Everything is but an image of eternal inconstancy. The laws of conservation of mass and energy, of entropy—all are dualistic "idols." The belief in "constants" is the origin of all human tragi-comedies, of all unhappiness. Why do we not recognize the eternal constancy of inconstancy, which is so obvious? And why do we not see the Unifying Principle of Yin and Yang, which governs all inconstancy?

The Unifying Principle is the key to awareness that we are always in the Kingdom of the Seven Heavens, the first six of which are colonies of inconstancy, the seventh being Infinite and Eternal Constancy. When we know the constitution of these seven heavens and we understand the yin-yang key (also known as Absolute Justice), nothing in this relative and finite world is a mystery to us.

I would like to explain to you why there are "a thousand and one" methods of curing cancer, allergies, heart disease, and mental illness: *Because the method of cure relates to each individual and each individual is different, there are innumerable approaches.* This knowledge takes into account the infinite multiplicity of phenomena.

These innumerable methods can be divided into two categories, symptomatic and fundamental. The latter approach is efficacious, whereas the former provides difficult and more temporary relief.

While the fundamental method (establishing a normal human balance) is basically identical for all diseases, its applications are personal and result in *countless nuances and subtleties.*

Man is trying his best, though in vain, to discover a symptomatic cure for cancer. Thousands can be found, but all will be palliative and weak at best. Eventually, there will be no choice but to adopt the fundamental method.

Please understand two very important points: first, the so-called "incurable" or "chronic" diseases can be cured through application of the ancient philosophy-medicine of the Far East, either as moral teaching, as dialectical diet, or both; and second, that you must study the dialectical and practical philosophy if you want to procure deep understanding of its medical, moral, and dietetic applications (which combine to produce its curative powers). This philosophy is interesting and extremely useful judging all ideas and action. With it, you can transform all unhappiness into happiness, all difficulty into joy, all sadness into gratitude, all "evil" into "good," all poverty into wealth, all sickness into health, all ugliness into beauty, all ignorance into wisdom, all weakness into force—and vice versa.

Have I succeeded in clarifying these two points? Have you grasped the first one? And the second? Perhaps you can see it, at least conceptually—but I do not count on you. It is perhaps a little too hard for you, my dear civilized friends—a conclusion I have regretfully reached after having tried so hard with you for so many years. And to add to the problem, you are educated! But, for the time being, I would be glad if only a handful in every country were to take interest in these studies.

It is difficult, this dialectical and paradoxical philosophy. Its conception of the world differs from your own. But why so difficult? Because of its simplicity! There are but two antagonistic concepts, Yin and Yang. That is all. But you must *apply* this unifying polar principle to your daily life. And while you may find this very embarrassing, it will also prove extremely interesting.

Since its revolutionary beginnings in the 17th century, modern science has progressed with giant strides. Francis Bacon violently attacked the four idols of the Tribe, the Cave, the Marketplace, and the Theater. Experimental science began. Positivism followed. The theory of Copernicus upset our classical view of the world. Then came mechanism, experimental medicine, and pragmatism, all of which required observation, description, experimentation, objective precision, and exactitude. Science ramified. Specialties and experts abounded. Finally, we have witnessed the death of the atomic concept and the beginning of transmutation, cybernetics, sputniks, and the production of 95,000 hydrogen bombs. Uncertainty and fear predominate. Where is our scientific and technical civilization headed?

This is another example of the inconstancy of our finite, relative world. Soon we will see either a catastrophe spelling the end of all mankind or the birth of a brand new world—an era of man after the animal era. Heretofore, all changes have been materialistic, sensorial, sentimental, physical, chemical, intellectual, economic, and technical—but not at all *human*. Now scientific and technical changes have reached a dead end, and a new and totally unknown avenue opens before us, leading to the development of man's judgment.

All our behavior depends on judgment—madness or sanity, war or peace, happiness or unhappiness. But there are seven stages of judgment: mechanical, sensory, sentimental, intellectual, social, philosophical, and supreme. The judgment responsible for scientific and technical civilization is limited to the first or second stage, mechanical or sensory. We must now listen to higher sounds.

The physical, economic, and technical revolution is greatly advanced. We have been proceeding at a fantastic speed. Why not also in a new philosophical and ethical direction? The question is only how.

It is a most important question.

Let us utilize the compass of Yin and Yang. This practical, dialectical logic, a universal logic, is sufficient. (However, do not confuse this instrument, so simple that anyone can manufacture and handle it easily, with the deified authority of Aristotle or the Bible.)

The scientific and technical civilization, which is in the process of collapsing, will change its direction once it has been supplied with this compass: Yin-Yang, and will very probably achieve an unprecedented revolution a thousand times more upsetting—because of its fundamental nature—than that provoked by Copernicus' theory. The science and techniques of today are dualistic and belong to the system of Ptolemy. They are exclusive, physical, and chemical. They are ignorant of life, memory, thought, spirit, matter, electricity, and magnetism. Above all, they are not aware of Oneness: Infinite Happiness, Freedom, and Justice. They are blinded by nuclear walls.

Science and technology have been advancing after the manner of Cook, Drake, and Christopher Columbus, i.e. groping blindly through unknown geography. To rebuild the scientific and technical civilization, we must make use of the Unifying Principle, the compass that is indispensable for navigation towards the new world of lasting peace and joyfulness.

But do not be afraid if there are few who listen to you and follow you. There are seven stages of judgment, and the lower the judgment, the greater the number of adherents.

The bigger the front, the bigger the back.

In like manner, if cancer is the most "incurable" disease, it is also the most "curable," the easiest to conquer if you seek its cause, which lies within you. Introspection will teach you how you produced it. If you discover the mechanism, you can then change the orientation of your ever-darkening civilization. In this sense, cancer can serve as your savior!

"An eye for an eye and a tooth for a tooth."

"Ten thousand grains for one grain."

The attitude represented by "An eye for an eye, a tooth for a tooth," is traceable to the infantile and savage mentality that lies at the heart of symptomatic medicine. It is a mentality full of hostility and curses. Its habitat is Hell.

But the philosophy and biology of the Far East proclaim: "Return ten thousand grains for one grain." In practical applications, one grain *does* yield about 10,000 grains. This is the fundamental law of biology. So, if you are rendered a one-minute favor, return a 10,000-

minute favor as a proper expression of your joy. If your benefactor is dead, return what you owe to his relatives. If your eye is pulled out, withdraw and ask yourself what was the cause of such cruelty. If the fault lies in the other's incomprehension, seek a way to save him through graceful behavior. If you cannot convince him gracefully, it is your own fault. Then, after you have transformed your enemy into your benefactor, look for 10,000 similar persons and transform them as well.

Remember, however, that in nature there is no such incomprehension. In nature, it is *always you who is wrong. It is your own fault.* If you become the prey of cancer, allergy, or any other disease, look before anything else to yourself. Find your errors, correct them, and then teach 10,000 people what you have discovered concerning disease.

"Ten thousand grains for one grain" is the expression of a deep mentality full of infinite gratitude, infinite joy. Peace can be found in its practice.

"Do not resist, even evil. If someone strikes you on the right cheek, turn to him also the left." This beautiful advice is difficult to practice because of low judgment restricted to the sensory or sentimental level. Our Far Eastern philosophy teaches, "If somebody wishes to strike or kill you, it is your own fault, because you yourself have angered him." Arguments and protests are worthless. Humbly ask forgiveness, then withdraw so that your presence may not irritate him even more. Try to find out how to behave in order to win his love, understanding, and gratitude. If he loves you, he will accept everything you say and will give you all he owns instead of hitting or killing you. Everything depends on a graceful approach. You must learn how "to convince without speaking" and "how to conquer without fighting."

Our philosophy also teaches that no enemy or evildoer exists in this world—nature and human society included. There is only misunderstanding, incomprehension, or awkward behavior.

Such is my interpretation of the words, "Love your enemy and pray for those who persecute you." This principle's biological and physiological counterparts are the foundation-stones of Oriental medicine, whereas it seems to me that "civilized" symptomatic medicine is the opposite; it curses and condemns, remaining a sworn enemy of disease to the bitter end.

Emotional exclusiveness is Hell itself. If you kill your antagonist, you lose, at that very instant, all hope of victory. You can no longer be the "winner," because the "loser" has ceased to exist. Or perhaps another antagonist will appear, this time defeating *you*. Vengeance is spontaneous. The first becomes the last. Victory is defeat. Everything is paradoxical in this relative world.

"Life is death," said Claude Bernard. He could have meant either that life leads inevitably to death or that life and death are two names for one and the same mystery. Is death the true identity of life? What do *you* think?

Oriental philosophy exhibits a panoramic view of the Infinite Universe and teaches that Life is eternal, that Life means to exist, and that the idea of "death" is simply an illusion. Death never exists. Death is a fiction created by a man bound in fear through mental blindness—clouded judgment. Only he who is afraid sees "enemies" and "death."

The practical and dialectical universal philosophy teaches how to live a long, amusing, and beautiful life—without fear of *anything*.

The Order of the Universe and the Unifying Principle

I. The Order of the Universe: *Seven Dynamic Universal Principles Which Describe the Relative World and its Relationship to the Infinite Universe (Oneness)*

1. All visible and invisible phenomena are manifestations of Oneness.

2. All visible and invisible phenomena are different from all others.

3. All visible and invisible phenomena are constantly changing.

4. All visible and invisible phenomena have a beginning and an end.

5. All visible and invisible phenomena have a front and a back.

6. The bigger the front, the bigger the back.

7. All antagonisms are complimentary.

II. The Unifying Principle: *Twelve Dynamic Universal Theorems Which Describe the Creation and Functioning of the Relative World*

1. Oneness (infinite expansion) continuously manifests itself, at all points and moments, as divisions of itself, which create 2 forces: centrifugality (expansiveness) and centripetality (contractiveness).

2. Let us call centrifugality "Yin" and centripetality "Yang."

3. Yin and Yang are constantly changing into each other.

4. At the extremes of development, Yin produces or becomes Yang and Yang produces or becomes Yin.

5. Yin attracts Yang and Yang attracts Yin.

6. The force of attraction between Yin and Yang is greater when the difference between them is greater, and smaller when it is smaller.

7. Yin repels Yin and Yang repels Yang.

8. The force of repulsion between Yin and Yang is smaller when the difference between them is greater, and greater when it is smaller.

9. Yin and Yang, combined in an infinite variety of proportions, produce energy and all other visible and invisible phenomena.

10. No phenomenon is only yin or only yang; all phenomenon are composed of both Yin and Yang.

11. No phenomenon is balanced; all phenomena are composed of unequal proportions of Yin and Yang.

12. All phenomena are yang at the center and yin at the surface.

"One produces two, and two produces three," said Lao Tzu. The "three" of his saying represents all that exists in this relative world (after Oneness divides, creating the polarity of *twoness*: Yin and Yang). Succeeding divisions continuously produce an infinite variety of phenomena. Where one force meets another (Yin and Yang meet), spirals form, thus producing more and more phenomena. This process is repeated endlessly, everywhere, all the time.

Yin is centrifugality: the force of expansion, dilation, and diffusion. Yang is centripetality: the force of contraction, constriction, and cohesion.

Yang produces heat, light, infra-red radiation, activity, dryness, density, hardness. Yin produces cold, darkness, ultra-violet radiation, passivity, wetness, lightness, and softness.

To say that something is "yang" means that its Yang (centripetal force) exceeds its Yin (centrifugal force), the reverse being true when we speak of something as "yin." For example, compared to woman, man is more active, compact, and hard. His flesh is actually brittle compared to that of a woman. Also, the percentage of red blood cells in his blood is higher. These factors (as well as many others) are all indicative of the fact that Yang (centripetal force) is greater in men than in women.

The Unifying Principle of Yin and Yang is nothing more or less than the law of Change, basis of the great religions of man. We see it in operation every day of our lives, but are often unaware of it. Night becomes day. sickness becomes health. Ignorance becomes wisdom... *And all vice versa.* If Yin did not become Yang, then what would? If schoolboys were learned, how could they be taught? Such is the mechanism of Absolute Justice: the yin-yang law, which governs all phenomena, visible and invisible.

The Common Cold

The common cold, the existence of which has been recognized since the early days of medicine, cannot as yet be cured. Modern symptomatic medicine in all its glory and pride can do no more than rebaptize it "general allergy." This word "allergy," a magic invention that explains nothing, discloses the ignorance, arrogance, and irresponsibility of scientific doctors throughout the centuries.

Recently, the United States government decided to spend 20 million dollars in the development of a vaccine against the common cold. Is it not ridiculous that such an enormous amount should be spent in search of a remedy that can only be symptomatic and palliative, especially in view of the fact that so many pharmaceutical, medical, and surgical inventions of the past, praised on first appearance, have turned out so often to be of questionable value at best? And if success is attained in the attempt to develop a vaccine for the 1,100,000 Americans who are afflicted daily with common colds, then will not something have to be done for sufferers of hay fever, whose numbers annually reach 30,000,000?

And this is only the beginning. President Eisenhower declared during a session of the 1954 Congress that "50 million Americans living today will die from heart disease," and that, according to official statistics, 128 million Americans suffer from chronic ailments. How many vaccines will have to be invented to complete the preposterous journey begun by Jenner and Pasteur? Is it not a vicious circle that produces more and more "marvelous" suppressants of an ever-growing army of symptoms?

105

Although the common cold has been renamed "allergy," it still exists and is even growing more prevalent. Strangely enough, no living species suffers from it anywhere near as much as man does; tigers, elephants, birds, and insects are not affected by it, nor are fish, worms, or grass. They all survive without colds and without central heating or warm clothing stolen in the form of wool and furs from other animals.

Why does symptomatic medicine not search instead for the mechanism of immunity exhibited by animals, birds, fish, and insects? Alas! When man thinks of them, it is only with the idea of killing them.

"If I must kill to defend myself," Gandhi said, "I prefer to be killed." All his life he deplored the fact that he found it impossible to abandon the use of goat's milk—in other words, to live without exploiting other animals.

To kill other living beings is to kill oneself. To exploit other living beings, to live as a virtual slave-owner, is also suicide. By surviving parasitically, one suppresses and allows to atrophy one's own creativity and productivity, which (according to Vedanta philosophy) are the essence of life itself. Modern, civilized man, so continual an exploiter of other animals including his own species, contracts more and more colds despite a yearly consumption of one thousand *tons* of aspirin in the United States alone.

But a cold cannot be defined as only a momentary ailment and the loss of a certain number of working days. For each such illness, we must pay a very high price in the form of hardening of the arteries and body tissues.

According to the Unifying Principle of Science and Philosophy of the Far East, the cause of a cold is general yinnization. We consume too much yin food, i.e. food rich in vitamin C, potassium, calcium, phosphorous, water, etc., and do not establish a normal yin-yang balance in our bodies. Instead of reestablishing correct yin-yang proportions in our diet, which would cure the *cause* of the disease, we ingest extremely yin drugs that eliminate *symptoms* (by paralyzing the ortho-sympathetic nervous system), and consequently bring about a considerably worsened condition.

Modern medicine exhibits no real concern for the causes of disease. It is *totally ignorant* of the cause of the common cold and, in fact, does not even search for it. Its prime concern is palliative treatment that will suppress a patient's symptoms. It is not even bothered by the fact that its search for a symptomatic remedy has proved fruitless.

Why, instead of looking for a fundamental, unifying and permanent solution to the problems of disease, does official medicine prefer an endless series of symptomatic, palliative, and temporary recipes? My conclusion is that the source of this failure is man's own dualism or separatism, diversely manifested in the oppositions of spiritualism-materialism, selfishness-altruism, science-philosophy, God-man, body-soul, *ad infinitum*. And from what source does such dualism spring? From nothing less than a very real sclerosis, *the death of brain cells.*

The "precision instrument" of modern civilization—science—is blind; its faculties of judgment are still impaired. (Without a practical technique, philosophy becomes useless, while at the same time a technique without a guiding principle is absurd and often dangerous. The best proof of this is the danger under which the whole of humanity lives today—nuclear annihilation.)

Monism is man's universal compass or direction-finder, pointing the way toward awareness of Eternal Happiness, Infinite Liberty, and Absolute Justice. But one should cautiously avoid equating it with rule of the majority, freedom by constitution, or legal concepts of "justice."

Today, we are witnessing the dramatic conclusion of all classic authority, the end of belief in the experimental techniques of August Comte, in the empirical approach of Darwin, the Cartesian philosophy of Kant, the theories of formal logic, atomism, and economic interchange.

Undoubtedly, Comte as well as other thinkers of the 18th century were wrong in predicting that the oppressive, conventional power of the deformed and mummified Catholic Church would soon be overthrown. Several centuries before Comte, Martin Luther, and Erasmus of Rotterdam had rebelled. Yet, even today, Catholicism rests secure in its dominion, and Protestantism itself has degenerated into another form of religion no less oppressive and reactionary. Moreover, at the end of his life, Comte himself turned toward "religion," just as Newton had done earlier.

Fortunately, Louis Kervran appeared at this critical moment in history to open new horizons of endless prospect through the infinitesimal windows of biological transmutation. His discovery not only terminates classical chemistry but also buries traditional scientific thought. His book, *Biological Transmutations*, contains a full explanation of his ideas.

Now science has reached an age in which it is being transmuted into philosophy. But "...modern science still belongs to the stone age," states Rachel Carson in her book, *Silent Spring*. And all who have read or listened to Kervran will agree. What, then, can we expect, philosophically speaking, of a science that has not yet developed beyond its "Neanderthal Age"? Could it conceivably grow and mature to a point where it might guarantee us awareness of Infinite Liberty, Eternal Happiness, and Absolute Justice? However generous we might wish to be, we cannot spare the thousands of years necessary to fulfill such a hope.

But, there is another way—the way of the Unifying Principle of science and philosophy of the Far East with its dialectics of Yin and Yang. This polarizable monistic principle was introduced in my first book in French, written about thirty-five years ago under the roofs of Paris when I was a poor student. Let us examine what it can bring us.

According to the theory of polarizable monism, we can classify into two antagonistic and complementary categories—Yin and Yang—not only all agricultural and industrial insecticides, but also thousands of commercial, sanitary, alimentary, biological, and physiological products.

Our health and vitality depend on the simultaneous introduction of yin foods and yang foods in proportions that will lead to the establishment of a normal human balance. Yin foods only, or yang foods only, lead to death. Unbalanced (abnormal) proportions of yin and yang foods result in disease, pain, unhappiness, crime, every manner of misery and difficulty and, to crown it all, nuclear war, the greatest of all diseases, posing a threat to the very existence of mankind.

The group of chemical elements with yang characteristics is composed of hydrogen (H), carbon (C), lithium (Li), sodium (Na), and arsenic (As). At the forefront of the yin group stands oxygen (O); then come nitrogen (N), potassium (K), phosphorus (P), and the vast majority of all other chemical elements. In my aforementioned book, *The Unique Principle: The Philosophy of Macrobiotics*, I explained the spectroscopic basis of this classification of chemical elements.

Biologists know that life on earth cannot exist without sodium *and* potassium. All living beings contain both—the proportion, however, varying with the characteristics of each species, its birth, and its way of living. Although some few species with very simple structures do live without these elements, such species still require a combination of two main elements (for instance H and O or C and O) in a relationship of yin and yang opposition.

If Yin becomes absolutely dominant in the constitution of a living being, such a being will disappear. The same result follows absolute dominance of Yang. Insuring a balanced proportion between Yin and Yang is of utmost importance. Bearing that in mind, we can assert that *there is no poison in nature*, only a lack of harmony, an improper balance between Yin and Yang (centrifugality and centripetality).

An organism with a stable constitution will be able to absorb and neutralize any unbalanced product—up to a certain point. In fact, we can even extend this theory to its ultimate by saying that healthy organisms can absorb and neutralize *any* poison. The historic case of the monk Rasputin is an example of this capacity pushed to the extreme.

In their actions as well, men exhibit opposing tendencies that can also be classified as yin or yang. When faced with a problem such as, for example, a constitutional disease, some men react with fear. Gradually or quickly, depending on the individual, this *fear* (yin) evolves into *hostility* (yang), which is expressed in violent attacks aimed at total suppression of symptoms. The cause, generally ignored, soon finds other means of externalizing itself. Thus, a chain of summary acts of violence disturbs and deteriorates the internal environment and, if unchecked, leads to death. Infernal prospect: nuclear war is the global equivalent of man's fear-inspired brutalization of himself.

Other men react to the appearance of disease with surprise rather than fear. They are driven to practice self-reflection and criticism in order to discover the cause, which is always ignorance of natural law. This search is facilitated by fasting and meditation, which lead to development of clear judgment, culminating in peace.

The first of these two attitudes epitomizes the way of life of a yang nation, whereas the second is that of a yin nation. Western civilization developed along former lines while Eastern civilization chose the latter road. Whether we are concerned with "biocide" resulting from chemical effluents or with the threat of nuclear annihilation, we are dealing with consequences of the first mentality.

The dualism of science cannot, of course, synthesize an overall concept of the universe. However, at present, a profound effort is being made the world over to develop a philosophy that will integrate all knowledge, including that of science. At this very moment, a dozen or more groups are working toward this goal in Japan alone. The death of Comte's theory is confirmed. Science today strives to become philosophy.

In the United States, Professor Herbert Ratner, a specialist in disease prevention and general hygiene, has recently shown that America is the richest nation—in terms not only of money but also in terms of sick people. Each day 1,100,000 citizens are afflicted with colds, while at the same time the nation holds first place in its exaggerated recourse to vaccination, surgery, medication, and drugs.

"Why are we the most miserable country in the world as far as health is concerned?" asks Professor Ratner. He concludes, "...because we lack a philosophy."

After all, science is but an instrument, a sensory technique for perceiving, experimenting with, and describing what is happening in this world of relativity. But Life is infinitely larger than science. In fact, it is the Infinite, of which our world is only an *infinitesimal geometric point*.

Life offers a double aspect, the "visible" matter of the world of relativity and the "invisible" that creates it. The visible always springs from the invisible.

"Matter comes from non-matter, and energy is continuously created from nowhere," concluded Professor P. W. Bridgman, before pessimistically abandoning his lifelong scientific researches and committing suicide at the age of seventy-nine.

Today, the existence of man is threatened by chemical "biocide" and nuclear war. Why this double danger unprecedented in the entire course of human history?

Our answer is simple. These threats are but two of the symptoms of a more fundamentally deadly universal disease, a disease of judgment. Man has been blinded during the past few centuries, intoxicated and paralyzed by chemical, symptomatic, and industrialized medicine, which is itself the product of so-called "formal" (dualistic) logic.

Appendix Three

Beyond Miracles

Those who practice macrobiotics for years, or who have grown up in its tutelage, possess great spiritual strength—what less fortunate people might consider "miraculous powers." But, actually, the word "miracle" is limited to the vocabularies of those who do not understand the Order of the Universe. Another commonly misused word, "Justice," serves macrobiotics in designating the constitution of the Order of the Universe and the dialectical principle of its change. These key words, "miracle" and "Justice" (as they are applied in ordinary conversation today), reveal profound misunderstanding.

Those who believe in miracles, who believe in the irrational, and who refuse to solve mysteries condemn themselves to the second or third level of judgment—sensory or sentimental.

Originally, empirical science belonged to the fourth, or intellectual level, where miracles are not believed in. But, as long as scientists credit a fiction such as "$E=mc^2$," they bear resemblance to naive "miracle-watchers." Strangely enough, many in the field of science employ only sensory judgment, the second level, evincing a kind of professional bigotry. Most scientific laws belong to a level that falls short of even Einstein's achievement—the fantastic hypotheses of Newton and Lavoisier and the thermophysics of Carnot, for example. Lechatellier's law* is a very rare exception, as is the law of asymmetry (which Pasteur lightly touched). If these laws had been

---

*In any system at equilibrium, any change in conditions results in a shift of equilibrium in a direction that will partially nullify the change.

perfected and unified, justice, truth, and the principle of Yin-Yang, which governs the universe, would have come closer to being understood. Other partial discoveries of this Order have been made, but as is natural with people concerned only with visible reality, nothing much has come of them.

Nevertheless, our disappointment might be somewhat premature because, as a result of the law "the bigger the front, the bigger the back," intelligent, sincere inquirers into the nature of the invisible world must certainly exist. Have there not been Goethe, Samuel Butler, Pierre Louys, and Elisee Reclus?

Much more extraordinary than miracles are: (1) The tremendous construction known as "the universe;" science hasn't even a glimmer of its size; after all, to science, that which cannot be directly perceived must be non-existent. (2) Perpetual transmutations, the Infinite Universe fostering all possible changes for each of its units and in each of its parts at fantastic and ever-varying speed. (3) The Unifying Principle, we can explain these changes and transmutations. (4) Rapidity: In this Endless Universe of billions upon billions of solar systems, each maintains its own orbit while moving with extraordinary velocity.

> The heavens themselves, the planets, and this center
> Observe degree, priority, and rank,
> Regularity, course, proportion, season, form,
> Attribute and custom, all in unvarying order.
> Shakespeare's *Troilus and Cressida*
> Act I, Scene III

(5) Life, which appeared in this heaven among these billions and billions of heavens! Is this not the greatest of all miracles?

"Our science is still a baby in the Stone Age," wrote Rachel Carson in *Silent Spring*. And this science-child knows nothing of the history, character, and function of the earth, its so-called mother. The joy of discovering the approximately 92 different elements failed to last, for these elements have disappeared like a mist, metamorphosing into a frail drop of dew called "sub-atomic particles." In one stroke, they have been changed into yin electricity and yang electricity. Has science lost its reason for existence? The visible world is finished. The invisible world has spectacularly revealed itself. Faced with this discovery, science holds its breath. Meanwhile, Life goes on and on, ceaselessly. Lovely colors appear in flowers, and trees deliver delicious fruit. The great sphere of earth produces proteins and fats, carbohydrates, vitamins, enzymes, and minerals. Plankton, fish, birds, and animals arise from the womb of earth in a continually advancing evolution! Oh! What a miracle!

(6) There is still a greater miracle—memory. Undoubtedly, one of the major achievements of the age of technology has been the computer, a machine that can do the work of several thousand intellectuals and a few million mathematicians. It is creating an industrial revolution. Yet, the human brain—which is one thousandth the size of the largest cybernetic machines—has a memory that is billions of times greater; is endowed with imagination, intuition, judgment, and will; and is capable of understanding peace, liberty, justice, happiness, health, beauty, and even love. Clearly, it is the greatest miracle!

All that science has discovered in the visible world is only a speck, a mere grain of sand on the limitless beach of the Infinite Universe. How ridiculous of humanity to have followed science with such trusting, cow-like docility!

(7) Science is undergoing a rebirth. This constitutes the seventh miracle. Having despaired when the visible world vanished, science is in the process of putting an end to its own misery. But one of its fifteen billion brain cells still functions: Kervran is his name. Yin (science) has produced yang (Kervran).

Kervran opened his eyes. He rose. He began to walk, surveying the new world. Observing carefully for more than thirty years, he heard the oracle of transmutation. In our present social milieu, it is practically impossible for him to be recognized by science. What he has seen is almost beyond belief, so much so that he himself at first doubted his vision. For thirty years, he chose to remain silent, re-examining the mechanism he had discovered, pinching himself to make sure it wasn't a dream.

At the same time, another miracle was occurring. Another man, born six thousand miles away, was looking for a Westerner who could understand the world of invisibility. After great difficulty, he finally found Kervran—two years ago at the age of sixty-eight. The bigger the front, the bigger the back: the joy of that old yellow man was very great indeed!

"You have opened the gates through which humanity can escape the sealed, small world of visibility. Before mankind stretches the magnificent prospect of becoming aware of the invisible world. Your discoveries are without precedent in the history of science!"

Did the two foreigners who met each other for the first time, after sixty and sixty-eight years of life on earth, understand one another? This would be an indication of a starting point for a true re-birth of science, which I hope for with all my heart.

But, there are still more extraordinary miracles. How tragic it is that those whose eyes are veiled cannot see them. It is as if they have been given tickets for the theater and sit numbly before a darkened screen while he whose judgment is unveiled perceives a fascinating extravaganza that lasts not a mere two or three hours, but five years, ten years, fifty years, and even billions of years. He is aware of Absolute Truth (Infinite Happiness).

Tickets for this universal spectacle are yours for the asking. Everything is free for those who have arrived at an understanding of the Order of the Infinite Universe and its constitutional principle: Yin and Yang.

The Seventh Condition of Health: Justice for Man

There are many things in this world that we "see without seeing," "hear without hearing," and "don't understand, even though we speak about them constantly." Justice is one of these.

Liberty, happiness, life, peace, eternity, health, harmony, beauty, truth—these as well as justice are objects of everyone's discussion and desire. Yet, it appears as though most people are intent upon finding the opposites of these in order to try to live "safely."

Slavery, unhappiness, death, war, disease, uncertainty, ugliness, lie, and law—all have their practitioners, professionals who specialize in the mass-manufacture or merchandising of these imitations of truth: salesmen of drugs, education, religion, ammunition, insurance, diplomas, technology, etc. The quests of science, philosophy, and revolution are equally misguided.

Both "visible" and "invisible" exist, the former measurable in the phenomena of the world we can see, the latter hidden beyond the reach of instruments. Some such as Democritus, Epicurus, Aristotle, Descartes, and Darwin decided that the "visible" constitutes the only true reality and that the invisible is non-existent. Their opponents claimed that the "invisible" is the true reality and that the "visible is only a shadow or illusion." Examples are philosophies such as Koku-u-zo-o (infinite expansion), Sunyata, and Vedanta, and individuals such as Lao Tzu, Gantama Buddha, Nagarjuna, Asanga, and Jesus Christ. (As with everything, one can distinguish two opposites that produce the drama of life in ever-changing, always-amusing scenes.)

After thousands of years, the proponents of "visibility" and "invisibility" began to despise and fight with one another. However, those who opted in favor of the "visible," denying the "invisible," were shocked to discover in the thirtieth year of the twentieth century that the "visible" was probably produced by the "invisible." The world of elements appeared to evolve from sub-atomic particles, and these seemed to come from "nothingness."

But those on the side of the "invisible" had so neglected the "visible" that they knew nothing, or next to nothing, about science. They stood by passively while researchers and technologists manhandled matter and pitched the world to the brink of destruction. Withholding their secrets, refusing to speak the language of science, they deprived mankind of the means of escape from its self-induced predicament.

And predicament it is. America, the Golden Dynasty, arch-proponent of the "visible," is lost in a storm of anger, uncertainty, and fear. Even its foremost scientists are aware of the precariousness of the times.

Some Orientals, sons of the civilization of "Bummei" (spirituality), were attracted by the civilization of "Butsumei" (materiality) and attempted to enlighten their adopted homeland. Sixty years ago, Kakuzo Okakura, author of *The Book of Tea*, and Etsu Sugimoto, author of *A Daughter of the Samurai*, published their stories about Far-Eastern civilization. During the same period, an American journalist named Lafcadio Hearn, who had married a Japanese girl and settled in her country, wrote about the Orient in an attempt to export its philosophy for the benefit of the Golden Dynasty. Unfortunately, like Okakura and Sugimoto, his judgment belonged to the third (sentimental) level. Thus, the lives and efforts of these people are commemorated in only a few works of literature, and their attempts produced no lasting effects.

Briefly synopsizing the Encyclopedia Americana, justice is defined as "something like happiness; it can never be attained by man." (This sort of judgment is to be expected from those who perceive only the "visible.")

Justice of man *is* attainable. But in order to attain it, we must first understand *Absolute Justice*.

Absolute Justice is not only the basis of justice for man; it is the basis of all existence; it is the source of all visible and invisible phenomena. Without it, we cannot live, not even for a second. It has been called by many names in the Orient, including "Amanomi-nakanonushi" (Master of the Universe), "Tao" or "Michi" (The Way of Life), "Tai-do-o" (The Big Road), "Taiko-o" (The Big Law), "Taik-yoku" (The Infinite One), "Taigi" (The Great Justice), and so forth. It is what I call The Order of the Universe. It is everywhere, all the time. If you understand it, you also understand and practice justice for man.

The kings of the world of "visibility" are matter, force, and war, while those of the world of "invisibility" are spirit, acceptance, and peace. The goal of the world of "visibility" is *relative* (satisfaction of desires), while that of the world of "invisibility" is *absolute* (aware-ness of Oneness). This is why the West and the East have so little in common.

One wise Western observer (Bergson), while journeying into his consciousness, noted that "The most striking characteristic of mod-ern Western science is its complete ignorance of Life." And what is Life? It is Absolute Justice!

Entering the Western Empire of the twentieth century, in which gold ruled supreme, I often felt as if I were one of the few remaining "primitives" of the world of invisibility, a comanchero, a Viking sur-vivor, or possibly even the last of the Mohicans. I was looked upon as an Oriental with spiritual or "mystical" abilities, but I considered this classification thoroughly misguided or even comical. Six years ago, during the first Far-Eastern philosophical (macrobiotic) meet-ing in France, there occurred a number of cures, and the people who gathered there came to be known as the "Miracles Group." That is how it all started. Following the "miracles," irrational people ap-peared like flies around a pot of jam. It seemed incredible that in this country of so-called "scientific civilization," so many helpless idol-seekers could have been spawned. But after all, I told myself, this was also the land of cartoons, cross-word puzzles, propaganda, and advertising. Here, television and the cinema prospered to the point where medicine, politics, the arts, and even religion used them as media for communication of public images. The *I Ching*, Zen, Tao, Hana (flower arrangement), Cha (tea ceremony), Haiku (seventeen-syllable poetry)—none admits of easy explication to the vast majority via public media. These are subjects that the teeth of "mass communication" cannot chew—impossible! And yet I am advised to speak on radio and television! There are actually people who call me "doctor." How annoying, sad, and pathetic! If Jesus had been called a gangster or murderer, how would he have felt?

I am a man who has amused himself his whole life long while enjoying a work that is diametrically opposed to that performed by so-called "doctors." What doctor would not be shocked to be called a murderer? I am even more humiliated to be called "doctor."

This is the sadness of an old man of the Far East who taught the secrets through application of which one can cure oneself of "incurable diseases" such as warts, rheumatism, lies, robbery, mental illness, and even war. I have spent my entire life without much sleep, without a home, enjoying only the smallest family pleasures, and now I am seventy years old! It is a very sad thing in this world to be considered at that stage of life as a specialist in symptomatic medicine.

Nevertheless, this does not matter. That I am considered a healer, a performer of miracles, or a magician, or that I am called "doctor"—well! after all, given I sell the "invisible world," it is only to be expected that I would be taken for a gangster or a swindler.

The seventh condition of health and happiness is the complete understanding and application of justice for men. This condition is far more important than the others—so much so that, if it is not fulfilled, achieving the other six is meaningless.

Not long ago, *Time* magazine related the case of a woman who had succeeded in lifting a car underneath which her son was pinned.

In the process, she slightly bruised one muscle—nothing more. This mysterious and unexpected power has often been called "spiritual." Nearly everyone has heard about some person who, during a fire or other serious emergency, was able to lift a load far heavier than normally possible, or about others who, upon finding faith, recovered from incurable ailments, or suddenly hit upon an answer they had been seeking in vain for years. This "faith power" or "spiritual power"—what is its source?

The miracles of Moses and Jesus have become fantasies, unbelievable marvels from the past. How typical of the Golden Dynasty! Yet, in the Far East, stories are told that are a thousand times more extraordinary. Sai-Yu-Ki (*The Monkey King*), an extremely long novel many hundreds of years old, is still read in China and Japan. Its translation into French required an effort of seventeen years. Sai-Yu-Ki—an original, amusing narration which conceals profound philosophical meaning—channels the reader's thoughts in the right direction without his being aware of it, teaching the pleasure and supreme joy of discovering the wonders of the Universe and the key to awareness of the fact that we are always in Paradise. It could be compared to *Aladdin's Lamp, Alice in Wonderland, Gulliver's Travels,* or the *Time Machine.* After reading it, one views the world of "visibility" as simplistic, superficial, and tasteless; one is stupefied by the idiocy and unimaginative banality of most movies and cartoons. Then, examining the idea of Maeterlinck, Uspenski, Gurdjief, Coue, Kinsey, Freud, or Swedenborg, one is struck by the superficiality of most Western mysticism and spirituality.

The works of Baudelaire, Mallarme, Valery, Rimbaud, and Poe, as well as those of a number of abstract painters, are very different from the symbolic works of the East. They appear to me to be escapist, as if the mentalities responsible for them were caught in desperation at the second level of judgment, suffocated by the "physical world" and frantic to reach the "invisible." The impression they convey is that life is a madhouse of tragic funerals, sickness, and disorder.

At about the age of fifty, I discovered that I could kill people with will-power alone, and I was startled. Without knowing I was endowed with such power, I actually killed two or three persons. I only wished to abandon, never to kill them, but they are dead. They disappeared like tailless kites. I felt very distinctly that it was I who was responsible.

Since then, I have completely devoted myself to the spread of this method of cure of body and soul: macrobiotics. Pursuing my goal, I have often forgotten to sleep and eat. Eventually, I arrived at the following conclusion: Nothing is *easier* to cure than so-called "incurable" disease, but nothing is *harder* to cure than patients themselves.

Later, I realized the importance, the enjoyment, and the suspense that come of struggling against such great difficulty, and I have given all my soul and all my strength to the endeavor. Time passed, the earth pursued its course, and I have reached the age of seventy. It is now, at this stage of my life, that I have come to know Absolute Justice, the Order of the Universe, the source of all spiritual power and "magical" capabilities.

But, awareness of Absolute Justice is not attainable overnight. Body and soul must be trained for thirty or even fifty years. One must climb the steepest snow-slick mountains, bitten by frost at every step of the way. If one is very strict, it is possible to arrive at the total understanding and practice of justice for man in only ten or twenty years. But, if one depends on a guide or an instructor, one will lose one's independence. Self-study is necessary to attain the ultimate goal. The following rules can serve as guideposts on the journey towards the comprehension and practice of justice for man.

(1) Never get angry. Accept everything with unlimited joy and gratitude, even if it be extremely humiliating, painful, or the cause of great inconvenience. Accept terrible misfortune or deep anxiety with ever growing thankfulness. Maintain yourself in such a condition that from morning till evening the words flowing out of your mouth reflect infinite gratitude.

(2) Never know fear. With a mental attitude that is fully prepared to accept whatever happens, seek what is horrible, repugnant,

or fraught with hardship.

(3) Never say, "I am tired; I am in trouble; it is difficult; what can I do?" or any similar expression.

(4) While eating anything, keep repeating, "What a joy, how delicious!"

(5) Sleep soundly and peacefully. Never dream, never move. Be content with four or five hours of sleep, awaking with a smile and at the designated time.

(6) Never forget anything—especially the spirit inherent in the maxim, "From one grain, ten thousand grains."

(7) Never lie to protect your "self."

(8) Be precise.

(9) Like everyone equally.

(10) Never doubt others.

(11) Attach yourself completely and solely to Absolute Justice, the Order of the Universe (change itself, the *only* constant).

(12) Discover and contemplate what being alive really means; understand that life is the most precious and greatest treasure in the world.

(13) Hour after hour, day after day, enjoy the pleasure and thrill of discovering the sublime Order of the Universe.

(14) Never work. (Never sell your time or your life for money.) Amuse and enjoy yourself to the end. Every day, all your days, live as a free man, the way the birds and the fish do in the skies and rivers.

(15) Live the principle "From one grain, ten thousand grains" by distributing joy and thankfulness to everyone you meet.

The Physiological Heart and the Psychological Heart

Existence depends upon the heart. As long as the heart keeps beating, we live; when it stops, the body ceases to exist physiologically. No engine can be compared to it. Our sentimental, intellectual, social, and ideological lives (joy, sadness, fear, confidence, knowledge, ignorance, etc.) depend on it.

Do we not often say "With all my heart," as if putting our greatest and most prized possession on the line?

But, in reality, we possess two hearts—two antagonistic hearts—and they are commonly confused: one is physiological, and the other is psychological. The former is a simple, faithful, honest, and potentially immortal mechanism, while the latter is extremely complicated, whimsical, sometimes dishonest, and sometimes brutal, cruel, and exclusive. (The potential immortality of our physiological heart and of all our cells and other organs has been established biologically by Dr. Alexis Carrel; see *Man the Unknown*.) All they require is an orderly environment, that is, suitable and appropriate nourishment.

Then why does the physiological heart die?

It is killed by our psychological heart, otherwise known as judgment. From the time of birth, our judgment grows towards the ultimate seventh stage called "Supreme Judgment." Biological and physiological education carry us through the intermediary stages. (I have given this education a more or less incomprehensible name: "macrobiotics." It is simply one application of the Unifying Principle Yin-Yang of the Philosophy and Science of the Far East.) Clouded judgment—and this is the secret—destroys the physiological heart.

In civilized countries, three plagues predominate: heart disease, cancer, and mental illness. One American out of four dies of heart disease, and throughout the world, several hundred million people must contend with its consequences day and night. Yet, those afflicted with mental illness far outnumber any other sufferers, contributing substantially to the social unrest and upheaval that beset modern man.

The psychological heart can, potentially, attain Supreme Judgment, but the physiological heart is limited by space and time.

Man must be fearless and adventurous; otherwise his life is not amusing. I admire fearlessness. But I deplore fearlessness in one who lacks Supreme Judgment (awareness of his true identity: Oneness). Nothing is easier than controlling the finite world by means of Supreme Judgment.

All heart ailments, including angina pectoralis, reflect a generalized condition of either vagotonia (dominance of the para-sympathetic nervous system) or sympathicotonia (dominance of the ortho-sympathetic). These diseases can be cured symptomatically with cortisone or chlorpromazine. (With macrobiotics, accurately understood and applied, one can cure them much more lastingly—in about one month.) And yet, deaths due to angina pectoralis have increased 70% in our times.

Perhaps you are one of those who has recovered from all manner of so-called "incurable" illnesses through macrobiotics. Not without risks and difficulties have I freely given you this means. But, if you *take* it freely, you are making a great mistake. You must study and understand fully *why* you had an "incurable" disease and *why* you were cured; read and re-read our publications several times; think and meditate; be a living example of a "miraculous" macrobiotic cure and teach the Unifying Principle to your children and neighbors. If you do not teach everyone you meet, if you fail to distribute this philosophy that guarantees awareness of Infinite Liberty, Eternal Happiness, and Absolute Justice, your cure will remain a debt, and sooner or later, you will forget this key to awareness of the Kingdom of the Seven Heavens. Or, if you introduce it as a mere symptomatic technique, you will fall ill again, seriously ill.

Appendix Six

The Kidneys: More than a Plumbing Fixture!

The kidney, the most precious and faithful of our organs, is the chemist of the body. In Far Eastern medicine, a direct relationship is said to exist between its functions and human sexual life, in this respect, it is our most important organ. But western medicine knows of no such relationship. Which view is correct?

Over nearly half a century, I have personally met thousands of patients. All, regardless of the type of disease, suffered with kidneys that were malfunctioning, blocked, or extremely exhausted. Yet, only a few had been diagnosed as suffering from kidney dysfunction. In relation to the kidneys, the other organs possess simpler structures and functions and are, therefore, subject to less difficulties: stomach, heart, liver, spleen, etc. The part played by the kidney is much more complex and delicate.

The kidney is the filtration system of blood, which carries oxygen and nourishment to the trillions of cells inhabiting the body and, at the same time, carries away impurities and waste products excreted by them. If we compare blood with the fuel of an automobile or airplane engine, we shall better understand the importance of the kidneys. In proportion to the gross mechanics of a motor, body activity occurs on a microscopic level. We know that if we mix foreign particles with fuel the car will stop or the plane will fall and crash. But our two small kidneys (3½ ounces each) filter and purify our blood night and day, even during our sleep, and are still more active when we work: several thousand quarts a day, several million quarts

a year, and this for fifty or even a hundred years—all with predict-
able regularity and constancy, without fatigue or failure.

The daily work of our kidneys can be compared to the effort
necessary to carry a 1000-quart vat to the top of the Alps. The kidney
is a giant-dwarf, a relentless worker, an accurate chemist who never
pauses for rest. From what source does it draw its endless energy?
Who controls the production of this precision instrument? Is it "au-
tomatic?" But who or what could be responsible for such "automa-
tism?" No professor can answer.

The kidney processes acids, impurities, and poisons, renewing
its constitution at every moment. How resistant! How small! How
creative! It is like a watch immersed in a chemically impure bath that
manages to work diligently without ever even having to be wound.
It is a very extreme act to abuse or destroy this living machine, this
giant-dwarf. Harming it even a little marks you as ungrateful, ignorant, brutal, cruel, and arrogant—ungrateful because you feel no joy
in owning such a treasure, and arrogant because arrogance and ignorance are synonyms, just as brutality and cruelty are. Your ignorance
is colossal. You are ignorant of all and All. No excuses. You love
your life but not Life. You do not understand what activates life. You
have no idea of its origin, mechanism, value, or significance. You are
in the dark as to exactly why and how you degrade it. You completely and utterly ignore Oneness, which imagines, realizes, creates, and
animates everything. You are deaf to the Voice that speaks through
these changing, ephemeral, and illusionary scenes. Thousands of
years ago, Oneness was called God. God had been discovered. But
alas! in the course of centuries, God has been forgotten or misunder-
stood, just as were Jesus, Buddha, and Lao Tzu.

Soul, Reason, Tao—the ear recognizes these words but nobody
knows their significance, their reality. Herein lies the misery of our
"knowledge."

Consider "thinkers" such as Camus and Sartre who declare
loudly and haughtily, "Life is absurd, completely absurd; we exist
without knowing why. We must, therefore, create our reason for being." What a deplorable declaration of ignorance! Existentialism is

a bomb built to destroy the Infinite, a pathetically finite contraption. One might as well hope to demolish New York, London, and Tokyo with one firecracker.

Nor is this all. So-called professional physicians claim to be able to repair or rejuvenate damaged or stagnating life. How? Without understanding Life? Or even life? Without understanding the Infinite Universe? Or even the finite universes? Are they not like ignorant and clumsy shoemakers who, because they have developed the cobbler's trade, believe they can create a human foot?

Such ignorance-arrogance governs and rules the modern world. Man is preparing himself for destruction, delighting in each new invention that turns out to be deadlier than his neighbor's. Thermonuclear bombs spring from the same mentality that produces medicines aimed at the destruction of germ-life.

But let us go back to our poor, ignorant, arrogant, ungrateful, simplistic, avaricious, brutal, and criminal patients who have ruined their marvelous kidneys.

Curing your kidneys, even of "incurable" diseases, is the easiest thing in the world. So strong that they can perform their delicate work for a hundred years or more, the kidneys are controlled and activated, day and night, by the autonomic nervous system. To heal yourself, observe these two steps:

(1) Learn the Order of the Infinite Universe, revealed through the finite universes, and know its Absolute Justice, the Unifying Principle of Yin and Yang. The biological and physiological application of this Unifying Principle (which any schoolboy can easily learn in an hour) is the medicine of the Far East. It is simply an instinctive art of life. Everything from monocellular organisms to the elephant lives by it without ever having attended medical school.

(2) Ponder the seven stages of judgment and learn to which stage(s) you belong. (Ed. note: Please see *The Atomic Age*—soon to be published—or, *The Macrobiotic*, vol. 10, no. 3.) I advise you with heartfelt and sentimental solicitude not to listen to simplistic professionals who recommend (for money) that you drink as much as possible: "This is a necessary and efficient method of flushing

out the kidneys," they claim. But many are those who know the destructiveness of this advice after wasting years and spending fortunes. These professionals have apparently forgotten everything they knew (learned in school) about the extraordinary function of the glomerules of Malphigi (extremely minute: four-thousandths of an inch thick), which are able to differentiate between water, sugar, and protein molecules.

How could anyone equate these marvelously delicate and precise microscopic mechanisms with big glass tubes—or city sewer systems? What rudeness! With such a mentality, is it any wonder they cannot see the mighty order of the Infinite Universe?

Appendix Seven

The Atom's Demise

Time passes. The atom, precious jewel praised by physicists, has had a short life-span of only twenty to thirty centuries. The indivisible unit of existence, jewel-toy and heirloom of the Atomic King, has broken apart and disappeared.

These last fifteen years have demonstrated to science that 99% of the universe is neither solid, liquid, nor gas. Stars, galaxies, and universes are made up largely of subatomic particles, which do not appear to follow any known scientific law. The Atomic King has, thanks to the strategies of Epicurus, Democritus, Plato, Aristotle, Locke, Descartes, Kant, and others, conquered the first sky, or *human* field; then the second heaven: the kingdom of *plants*; then the third sky: *elements*. But the Atomic King's reasoning and logic have lost all power before the entrance to the fourth heaven: sub-atomic particles. There, his travel-permit is no longer valid. He must obtain a new visa if he wishes to continue his voyage through the remaining three relative heavens.

So the three conquered skies have vanished, and the atomists have lost their "raison d'etre." Perhaps the next step will be their suicide together with the whole of humanity in one great atomic convulsion.

But "All visible and invisible phenomena have a front *and* a back." On the other side of the planet exist a people governed by a Unifying Queen who rules not only the fourth heaven (sub-atomic particles) but the fifth as well (energy). Her only ruler is the seventh heaven, "Shin" (Life, Eternity, Infinite Liberty, Absolute Justice).

This Unifying Queen is the vehicle or mother of all existence. She governs billions and billions of universes. She is the representative of Absolute Justice in the relative world. She produces, animates, and transmutes everything incessantly and forever.

Two thousand five hundred years after Lao Tzu, a representative of the Queen has been sent to the Western world in the midst of its preparations for the destruction of humanity and the earth, this infinitesimal planet in the Infinite Universe. The representative's mission is to distribute magic glasses that enable one to see the two hands of the all-producing Queen—in other words, opposites: beauty and ugliness, greatness and insignificance, strength and weakness, health and disease, happiness and unhappiness, etc. These magic glasses, called Yin and Yang, unmask the secrets of creation. With them one can transform unhappiness into happiness, ugliness into beauty, weakness into strength. The Queen's law is the Unifying Principle of all transmutation, fundamental basis of the I Ching or Book of Changes.

Three scientists, Crick, Watson and Wilkins, won the Nobel Prize for their discovery of the secret code of living matter: Yin and Yang in spiral form, the double-helix of the chromosome. But they completely ignored the most significant aspect of their discovery, Yin and Yang. Instead, they were looking for the "basic unit of matter"—just as the atomists had! Not only that, they sought the Infinite (Life) within the finite (life), *instead of vice versa.*

These three Nobel Prize winners finally discovered the important antagonism between sodium and potassium (again, Yin-Yang), which I had been explaining for fifty years as a bio-chemical application of the Unifying Principle.

Appendix Eight

Spirals

If you leaf through a book on crystallography, you see nothing but spirals in all shapes and sizes. Allow melted paraffin to crystallize, and it will form spirals. Egg white (albumen) when dried, spontaneously produces the natural spirals of protein. And, if you examine plastic material—polyethylene—under an electron-microscope, its squared spirals become apparent.

Everything in the world exists in spiral form—even you. You can see spirals at the root of the hair atop your cranium, on the inner flesh of your fingertips, and on the soles of your feet. The more complete your spirals are, the healthier you are—for which you may be thankful to your mother.

Using electron-microscopes, biologists have studied the structure of muscles, the uterus, and intestinal walls. All are in spirals of more or less varying complexity. Water escaping through any funnel whirls, the direction of the spiral depending on the hemisphere. If you have seen a group of children holding hands in a circle, you may have seen that their circle grows continually smaller; they have to back away from one another again and again. If you were to blindfold them, they would all cluster together in the center. Snails and shellfish possess spiral shapes. Leaves and seaweeds grow in spirals. Flies, having taken in some poisonous substance, whirl spirallically upon themselves before dying. Birds never land directly but descend to earth in great spirals. Planets travel spiralic orbits. Behind planes and cars spirals form; so the tail end is constructed in such a way as to take advantage of (or neutralize) these swirls.

All such spirals mimic the universal (logarithmic) spiral. The Romans, whose buildings stood square and stolid, were ignorant of this key to understanding the universe. (The Celts, however, did use spirals in their architecture.)

Centripetal spirals are always accompanied by centrifugal spirals. Through the centripetal spiral, things condense and solidify. Through the centrifugal spiral, things evaporate and are scattered into space.

Do you know of any centrifugal spirals?

What about typhoons?

Scientists have built an extremely powerful device—the cyclotron, which produces centrifugal spirals. That's the West for you; trying to fulfill its egocentric dreams by projecting its distorted view of Life on the rest of humanity, by building...another machine!

Some astronomers claim that the universe is in a state of expansion. This is true. But how? Why? Silence...they are unable to explain. Maintaining that all heavenly spirals are centrifugal and that all the planets came from the sun, they conclude that there must have been some fantastic explosion: the "Big Bang." But what exploded? This, one of the great "mysteries" of modern science, also remains unanswered.

In human life, there are two fundamental spirals: centripetal (yang) and centrifugal (yin), the former being the process of materialization of man by means of the seven stages of evolution, and the latter being the process of dematerialization or spiritualization by means of the seven stages of judgment. And while those who become rich and powerful can still accomplish this latter process, those who do start off with money and power and later reach awareness of Oneness (7th stage of spiritualization: Supreme Judgment) are rare, very rare.

I once saw a Western book on ethnography in which the evolution of man's social development was pictured in a great spiral. In the center stood the family; then came the village, towns, cities, states, and nations, all of civilization being positioned at the extreme limit of this expansion.

We can see a similar view in the spiral of the elements: Hydrogen is placed in the center and, as the spiral unfolds, increasingly heavier elements such as Helium, Lithium, etc. are added, the Uranium group being positioned at the end.

A third example of a centrifugal spiral is the radiation of atoms. The centrifugality of these spirals is obvious from the ferocious destructive capabilities of the atom bomb. Centripetality (Yang) suddenly becomes centrifugality (Yin). A terrible explosion occurs, and everything disperses in radioactive disintegration. (Aikido, which is also based on centrifugality, also generates great power.)

The entire universe is composed of spirals, which always appear as pairs. The yang centripetal spiral convolutes to a point of materialization, while its yin "spouse" unfolds in dematerialization (spiritualization). Churches, for example, are quiet, cold, and blueish (yin), accentuating the spiritual. If they were cheerful, warm, and red, you might be more inclined to dance than to pray while inside them.

Someday as you are leisurely walking near a riverbank, observe the many spirals forming there. Collisions between moving water and stones or branches form centripetal spirals. But, at the same time, their antagonistic yin spirals whirl through them. These two are front and back.

Everything exists in spiralic form. Consider water as it disappears into a sink; it whirls. This is a graphic example of the meeting of Yin and Yang in our everyday lives. How wonderful!

In the air surrounding a plane in flight or a moving automobile, countless such meetings occur, forming spiral after spiral.

An electron is neither a grain nor a particle; it is rather a current, a manifestation of the infinite expansion forming another spiral through the meeting of Yin and Yang. Toward the center of the spiral, energy gathers and accumulates, so that in the very center electrons form protons, which, in turn, become neutrons. (That the *negative* electron yields a *positive* proton is startling to the modern Western scientific mind. Yet, in history, such transformations are more or less taken for granted. Every great nation, for example, as Toynbee and others have observed, ends in insignificance, while those that were previously insignificant later rise to greatness.)

In formulating his "law" of "universal magnetism," Newton assumed that the space between heavenly bodies is empty. (He said, "It is absurd to consider space as being void;" nevertheless, he made his calculations on the basis of such an assumption!) What an enormous error! There is no emptiness—only infinite expansion. Democritus' theory that the universe is composed of "emptiness and atoms" must be firmly denied. If space is empty and the atom (as science has discovered) is non-existent, then what does exist? Nothing?

At the equator, the earth rotates at about 1,000 miles an hour, revolving around the sun at about 70,000 miles an hour, while the sun moves about the center of this galaxy at about the same speed, and the galaxy itself is also in flight. At these amazing speeds, how do we stay on the earth? According to Newton, the answer is "gravity." But what is gravity? No scientist has ever explained it; it has only been measured. The answer, according to my way thinking, is that "gravity" is a manifestation of the Infinite Expansion, which *pushes* everything on the surface of the earth towards its center. Electrons, as we have said, are not particles of matter; they are a current, a stream, which flows from the eternal source (Infinite Expansion) and comes to a stop in a form called "proton." Between electrons and protons are many other stops, called "subatomic particles." (Yukawa received the Nobel Prize for discovering the "neutrino," but now the neutrino has been denounced; it no longer receives official scientific approval. Thus, modern Western science now admits that Yukawa received his coveted Nobel Prize for expounding a lie.) Everything proceeds from electrons to protons, then "fades away."

Why is it difficult for modern scientists to understand that *negative* electrons become *positive* protons? By the same token, *poor men* are most suited to becoming *millionaires*. (If you see some who remain poor, it is their own fault.) It is the most *obscure* who become the most *famous*. (For example, Disraeli, whose birthday is still celebrated in England, was an immigrant, an insignificant Jew who came to London penniless and unknown.) The greatest men always come from the lowliest origins. Such is the mechanism of Absolute Justice: Yin becomes Yang, and Yang becomes Yin. Electrons become protons, planets become suns, night becomes day, poverty becomes wealth, unhappiness becomes happiness, sickness becomes health...and all vice versa.

Appendix Nine

Sexuality: The Daybreak of Life

The most difficult disease to cure is loss of sexuality. If man loses his masculinity and woman her femininity, life becomes unutterably sad. A life without passion, emotion, love, adventure, ambition, joy, treachery, jealousy, deception, struggle, or competition is like salt without taste or grain without sweetness. Such a life is cold, dark, and bleak.

Life is a passionate sonata played by the two invisible hands of Yin and Yang; even death is a fugue—or a nocturne.

Sexuality is the daybreak of life! *It is the basis of all existence—* the key to genesis. Even atoms, elementary and nuclear particles possess sexuality—in the form of attraction and so-called "binding force." All the more so for all living beings. (In man, sensorial love is the flower of sexuality.)

Love between stars and planets has been called, falsely, "universal magnetism." This notion (Newton's) became the basis of modern physics. Sexuality being the primordial Order of the Universe, all life depends upon it. Neither existentialism nor essentialism (nor any other view of Life) could have been born without it. In fact, all living beings, as well as inorganic atoms, stars, galaxies, and universes, possess sexuality. Everything with beginning and end moves in response to its forces.

In the Far East, there is a very beautiful story about love among stars. They charmingly meet once a year, every year. Imagine— heavenly love affairs! Orientals celebrate encounters between stars more gracefully than do Westerners in acknowledging Christmas and

Easter. On bamboo poles ranging in length from fifteen to thirty feet, rectangular pieces of paper in seven colors are aligned. On them are written the poems of young girls and women who dream of eternal love. The bamboo poles can be seen planted in front of every house, rich and poor alike, on the seventh evening of the seventh month of each, in hopes that the evening wind will carry these poetic prayers off to the far, far distant stars. Love is life!

There are seven stages of love: blind, sensory, sentimental, intellectual, social, ideological, and universal. With few exceptions, Westerners know only the blind and sensory levels and have never even heard of the seven words that describe the various stages of love. Very seldom does one meet a person endowed with love of the highest level (who accepts everything without question forever). It is this that I most deplore in the West. Every morning, newspapers tell of tragic love affairs—all blind, mechanical, sensory, sentimental, or social, all short-lived and culminating in murder, scandal, or suicide. Based on love of money, fame, beauty, knowledge, or power, they result in desperation. Although such ties can bind people powerfully, we should seek love of the higher levels—otherwise, our lives are like those of the lower animals who are *incapable* of the higher levels of love.

Why are there so many sexual tragedies in the world, today?

The answer, quite simply, is disease. Fully 75% of all "civilized" people suffer from dysfunction of the genital glands or organs! Sexual education, although highly advanced in the West as well as in Westernized countries, is based on sensory, sentimental, or intellectual judgment. Such education completely overlooks the biological, physiological, and logical training necessary to teach the seven stages of love and lead the student toward understanding of the Order of the Universe.

During recent years in Europe and the United States, I have examined hundreds of people tormented by sexual problems. I have seen cases of impotence; homosexuality; vaginal hemorrhages; hermaphrodites; morphological and psychological sexual abnormalities; women with no menstruations or with irregular, long, painful or foul-smelling menstruations; "frigid" women; women without sex appeal; and "masculine" women who protest, object, attack, growl, shout, and fight. Alfred de Musset, Albert Samain, and many other poets would today repent for having written their eulogies of the opposite sex. Could there still exist a Rosemonde Gerard to write a poem about eternal love? And would not Pierre Louys, author of "Astarte" (the eternal virgin), my favorite French poem, be startled to meet a barren young girl, a thirty- or even fifty-year old spinster?

There are numerous diseases of the genital glands and organs, and everyone suffering any chronic illness is also afflicted with some such trouble. This accounts for the high incidence of unsuccessful marriages and divorce in the West. Even the Catholic Church, *originally* a religion of tolerance, was compelled to outlaw divorce in order to protect the female. In Japan, on the contrary, there exists a Buddhist temple called "En-Kiri" (literally, marriage cutter), where any woman can rid herself of a cruel husband. Despite appearances, Far-Eastern society is feministic and acknowledges the superiority of woman on biological and physiological grounds. The mother is seen as creative, the father destructive. Woman never makes bloody wars, while the male is the "enfant terrible."

If the male grows effeminate and the female turns masculine— yang loses its yang qualities (especially its iron will) and yin loses its yin qualities (especially its grace and tolerance)—marriage ends in tragedy, marking the termination of one unit of humanity. On a larger scale, totaling the increasing numbers of such tragedies, we can foresee the potential decline and eventual obliteration of all human life.

On the subject of pathology—and since I am an "advocate of female supremacy"—let us first consider woman. Because she is superior to man, the appearance of body hair on women represents a true decline and the first symptom of a fatal disease for humanity. Women with hair on their feet have lost the natural characteristics of the more beautiful sex: all the more so for women with hairy arms, because the arm is more yin than the foot. A glance at the hairy feet of a woman gives goose-bumps to a Japanese male.

The difference between man and animal has been expressed biologically in the Japanese language. Man is a hairless creature, or "hito," while animals are "kedamono," (hairy). One advance marking man's evolution from animal stages was the loss of body hair over billions of years. Woman, being more evolved than man, has smooth, beautiful skin. And even though her skin is not covered with as much hair as a man's, a woman is more resistant to cold.

Women with hairy legs have destroyed or masculinized their sexual glands and are, in fact, no longer women. When all women have become hairy, the end of the world will be at hand. Such a state of affairs (an hermaphroditic existence) would be worse than hell, and would constitute a much greater misfortune than thermo-nuclear war because the latter, although destroying mankind, would at least be quick about it.

How can a woman be made beautiful? How can the Mother of Humanity by resurrected? This is one of my secrets. I give it, not for a thousand million dollars, but freely: macrobiotics! Specifically, an eating pattern very low in animal protein, which, therefore, eliminates hair in two or three weeks. It is unbelievable—it is black magic! See for yourself.

The human being is sexual; life is sexual; to be without sex means death. So it is that France, the country of love, of proper sexuality, attracts many Westerners to its capitol. Indeed, foreigners who in their own country never enjoyed passionate love, love that teaches the profound significance and joy of being, fall under her spell—especially in the springtime (yang). In their own country, love is almost non-existent. Four out of five men are desperate for sexual satisfaction, suffering a conjugal life they consider torturous. One out of ten thousand, or even a hundred thousand, really enjoys marriage.

Once upon a time, a very brave American came to France in search of eternal love. He was even prepared to remain in Paris for the rest of his life. His name was Henry Miller. Soon, however, he realized that Infinite Love, as well as the joys of unlimited sensorial love, were not to be found there, and he was disappointed. Everything struck him as relative, ephemeral, and illusory because he was looking for the Infinite and Absolute within the finite and relative world. Such quests always end in tragedy: waste of time, waste of life. And such is the magic of sexuality—it provides us with the most amusing tragi-comedies imaginable.

Science, too, looks for "K's" (constants). Until recently, the most sought-after constant has been the atom, the hopefully indivisible basic unit of matter. Lately, however, under the urging of nuclear physicists, this constant has "legally" changed its name to "sub-atomic particle." But, the idea that such elementary particles are "constant" is ridiculous.

Likewise, in this floating and inconstant world, this world of illusion, *the source of all human tragedy lies in the demand for change-lessness.* Our particular failure in the case of sexuality is blindness to the primordial polarization of the universe itself. Indeed, *the universe is sexual; it is not asexual. Sexuality permeates everything.*

It is impossible to progress from dualism to a monistic view of reality; the direction is backward. Rather must we begin, as does the Bible, with monism in order to explore the dualistic world. In Cartesian systems such as Teilhard de Chardin's, the starting point being dualistic, it is impossible to eventuate in a monism capable of unifying matter and non-matter, known and unknown, illusion and reality, or visible and invisible. Children of "visibility," such philosophers reject all that is invisible despite the fact that their great master, Descartes, discovered the "thinking ego," *which is invisible!* Memory, judgment, will, and faith—fundamentals of our existence—do exist and are knowable despite their *invisibility.*

The antagonistic but complementary (monistic) nature of sexuality is a great mystery to our Modern God, the scientist (who has replaced the omnipresent, omniscient, and omnipotent but outdated God of former times). All misfortunes, diseases, tragedies, problems, disasters, and crimes result from ignorance of sexuality and its law: dialectics.

Because as human beings we wish to lead ever happier, more exciting, and more amusing lives (otherwise, why bother?), we must contemplate the mighty Order of the Universe and its Unifying Principle of polarized monism. To assist in this contemplation is, or rather used to be, the only goal of the Church, but this has unfortunately been forgotten. First the Greek church, then the Roman, and finally the western Church are equally guilty of having become ritualistic, professional, and conventional.

Sexuality is the essential secret of life, of existence, of being, of adaptability. It consists of two forces—Yin and Yang—which are contradictory *and* complementary. Possessing this key, we can gain awareness of the fact that we are always, knowingly or not, in the Kingdom of Absolute Peace, Freedom, and Justice.

Man represents Yang, and woman represents Yin. Man is active, aggressive, destructive, greedy, and eager for possession. Woman is passive, receptive, creative, generous, and eager to be possessed. Man is wild; woman is refined. She is far superior to him biologically and physiologically.

Men want to love all women who are feminine. Women are happiest when they are attracted to, and dominated by, the most capable, adventurous, audacious, and ambitious man. A man who has neither ambition nor an adventurous spirit is a rotting, paltry being: a slave. Man and woman choose each other in accordance with a judgment that is influenced or governed, always and without exception, by the search for opposite traits. This is the yin-yang law of affinity ("The force of attraction between Yin and Yang is greater when the difference between them is greater, and smaller when it is smaller.")

Man's attraction to woman is most difficult to control and, therefore, also most exciting! The strong always love the weak, the fragile, and the innocent. The learned love the foolish, ignorant, and silly. Those who are destructive love those who are constructive, the rich love the poor, and so on. Such are the amusing, sometimes ridiculous, satisfactions of man.

But Eternal Happiness includes love *and* hate, strength *and* weakness, knowledge *and* ignorance, destruction *and* construction, wealth *and* poverty, health *and* sickness. So, in order to be strongly unified, a husband and wife must possess antagonistic qualities.

Life is paradoxical. All that is created is later destroyed. Eels lay millions of eggs, which are later eaten by other fish. Men produce billions of sperm cells, all except one of which die out before reaching the goal.

"But this doesn't make sense; it's not fair," you say.

"Wrong," I answer. Life is paradoxical. Everything possesses a double structure. "Fair is foul; and foul is fair." (Shakespeare) *To love and to hate are synonyms*. A courageous man does not know courage. Very often a man kills the woman he loves most.

These concepts may seem difficult to comprehend at first glance; but they are actually very simple because they are mere reflections of the two antagonistic forces that govern the world.

To love and be loved is to be engaging. To be the most learned and the most ignorant is to attain modesty. To be wealthy and a spendthrift is to be detached (in fact, such a person might be called the image of God).

First and foremost, learn the Unifying Principle, digest it, assimilate it, and use it in your daily life. Sit, for example, at the same table with your spouse and eat a meal containing balanced proportions of yin and yang food and drink (relative to your condition and environment). You will both become happier and happier. (If a woman wishes to become beautiful and happy, she must make herself more yin than her husband. Above all else, she should strongly avoid animal products, because most of them are so yang that they are unworthy of such a delicate constitution as woman's. Animal foods are more acceptable for a man, a wilder and rougher creature.

In effect, we are what we eat. Sexuality, the most primordial and beautiful quality in man, the flower of his existence, depends on diet. Cows—typical vegetarians—are peaceful, docile, and obedient. They spend their lives being exploited and finally wind up as beefsteak or clothes. Unconditionally obedient, as were Pavlov's dogs, they are less yang than man, who is normally very different from a domesticated animal.

If you eat only raw vegetables as do cows and are fed on the milk of those slave animals in your infancy, you will tend to become like a cow, and to spend your entire life being exploited as a "clerk," a "professional," or a public servant who faithfully serves his dicta-tor, "*Money*." Your judgment will remain at the blind or mechanical level, like that of a cow.

If you eat large amounts of animal products, your judgment will become increasingly animalistic.

Everyone eats, but few know how to eat. Only a person who eats in such a way as to achieve a normal human balance lives a happy life. Misfortune strikes those whose bodies and minds are not healthy. Such people often evidence sexual deviation as one among their many symptoms. In point of fact, homosexuality is quite com-mon in the West, perhaps a thousand times more so than in the East. Sexual deviation is the most miserable of diseases, and clouded judgment is its cause.

Sexual appetite is second only to appetite for food in man's gal-lery of desires. We live by appetite, an infinite gluttony that produces sexual longing. Controlling these twin appetites is extremely diffi-cult. He who understands the Order of the Universe and the Unifying Principle of Yin and Yang can do so if he wishes.

Consider the mechanical life of the industrious bee. Must man, his whole life long, also be content only to fill his stomach and sat-isfy his sexual needs? If you suffer from abnormal sexual desires, you are neither human nor animal. Homosexual and asexual beings are tragic, and Western literature is rife with them: *The Portrait of Dorian Gray* and the stories of the Marquis de Sade are only two examples.

You can cure sexual deviation with macrobiotics. By all means, enjoy love in the animal fashion, at the first stage of judgment, mechanical or blind. But develop yourself, your love, to the sec-ond (sensorial) level (which, however, always ends tragically, as is shown, for example, by de Maupassant). Then raise your love to the third (sentimental) level (which always ends in hallucination—see *The Biography of Stephan Sweig*). Hurry along, then, to reach in-tellectual love (as illustrated in the biographies of numerous scien-tists), social love (revolutionaries and reformers), and ideological love (philosophers). Finally, attain the seventh stage of judgment—Supreme, Infinite, Eternal Love where only endless happiness and infinite freedom are seen, felt, and known. This is the goal, and the result, of macrobiotics.

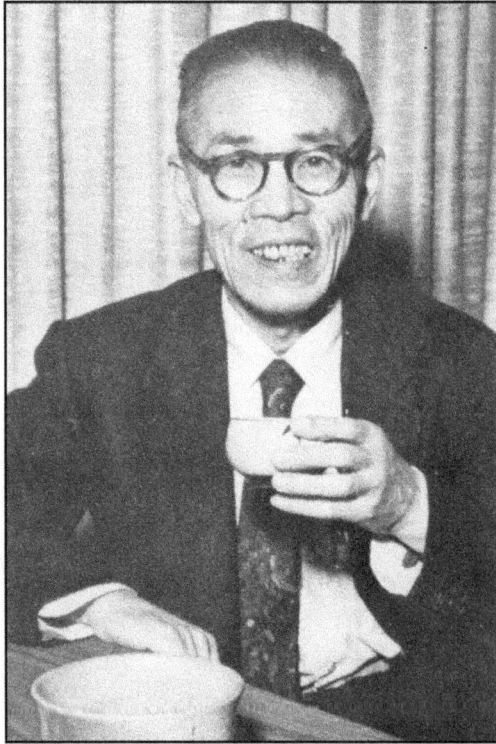

GEORGE OHSAWA

The Author

George Ohsawa (Yukikazu Sakurazawa) was born in Kyoto, the old capitol of Japan, on October 18, 1893.

He is the author of more than three hundred books, ten of which have been published in France since 1926. His work *A New Theory of Nutrition and Its Therapeutic Effect*, written and published in Japan in 1920, is in its seven-hundredth edition.

Thirty years of his life were spent introducing Oriental culture to Europe, while simultaneously interpreting the culture of the West for Japan. Among his many translations into Japanese are *Man, the Unknown* by Alexis Carrel and *The Meeting of East and West* by F. S. C. Northrup.

His passing on April 24, 1966 deeply saddened the countless individuals who are eternally indebted to him for having given to them of life itself. Their infinite gratitude is expressed in a continuation of the vital work he undertook and so ably pursued for more than fifty-four years.

A list of books by George Ohsawa and others on macrobiotics can be obtained from the George Ohsawa Macrobiotic Foundation, PO Box 3998, Chico, CA 95927-3998; 530-566-9765; fax 530-566-9768; *gomf@earthlink.net*. Or, visit *www.ohsawamacrobiotics.com*.